THE DAY MY HUSBAND was given his diagnosis of prostate cancer, his doctor gave us a copy of this book. He told both of us to read it prior to the upcoming visits my husband would have with the surgeon and radiation oncologist in the near future. The information in this book, and its question and answer format, made understanding what we were facing so much easier. It even provided a place to jot down our own questions and concerns to discuss with the doctors during upcoming appointments. As we tried to make a decision about treatment, we often referred to this book to verify that what we thought we understood was in fact correct, and to find answers to new questions that seemed to crop up as we tried to ready ourselves for "THE FIGHT," as we called it. Perhaps the doctor actually answered some of these questions during that first visit, but truthfully, "CANCER" was the only word either of us heard. Just one more reason it made sense to send us home with this book. My sincerest thanks to Dr. Pamela Ellsworth for writing it, and to our doctor for giving us a copy.

—Mary Stevens
LaGrange, KY

100 Questions & Answers About Prostate Cancer

FIFTH EDITION

Pamela Ellsworth

Professor of Urology University of
Central Florida College of Medicine
Orlando, FL

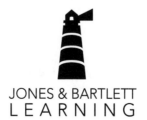

JONES & BARTLETT
LEARNING

World Headquarters
Jones & Bartlett Learning
5 Wall Street
Burlington, MA 01803
978-443-5000
info@jblearning.com
www.jblearning.com

Jones & Bartlett Learning books and products are available through most bookstores and online booksellers. To contact Jones & Bartlett Learning directly, call 800-832-0034, fax 978-443-8000, or visit our website, www.jblearning.com.

Production Credits

Director of Product Management: Amanda Martin
Product Manager: Teresa Reilly
Product Assistant: Christina Freitas
Product Assistant: Anna-Maria Forger
Production Manager: Daniel Stone
Marketing Manager: Lindsay White
Manufacturing and Inventory Control Supervisor: Amy Bacus

Composition: Miranda Design Studio, Inc.
Cover Design: Scott Moden
Rights & Media Specialist: Wes DeShano
Cover Image: © Tanya Constantine/ Blend Images/Getty Images
Printing and Binding: McNaughton & Gunn
Cover Printing: McNaughton & Gunn

ISBN: 978-1-284-15234-0

6048

Printed in the United States of America
22 21 20 19 18   10 9 8 7 6 5 4 3 2 1

Questions 1–10 describe the anatomy and function of the prostate, introduce the concept of prostate-specific antigen (PSA) testing, and discuss some of the potential warning signs of prostate cancer:

- What is the prostate gland and what does it do?
- Do women have a prostate gland and PSA?
- What are the signs and symptoms of an enlarged prostate (either cancer-related or benign)?

Questions 11–23 describe prostate cancer and address concerns about who is at risk for prostate cancer, including:

- What is prostate cancer?
- How common is prostate cancer?
- What are the risk factors for prostate cancer, and who is at risk? Is there anything that decreases the risk of developing prostate cancer?

Questions 24–40 discuss how to screen for and detect prostate cancer:

- How do you detect prostate cancer?
- What is prostate cancer screening?
- Will my insurance cover prostate cancer screening and treatment?

Questions 41–45 describe how cancer is "staged" so that an appropriate treatment can be determined:

- How does one know if the prostate cancer is confined to the prostate?
- How and why does one stage prostate cancer?
- What is a bone scan?

Introduction

If you're reading this book, you're probably concerned about your chances (or a loved one's) of getting prostate cancer—or you may even have been diagnosed with prostate cancer already. Like many people at risk for a disease like prostate cancer, you may wish to be proactive about your health—to read and learn about this disease so you understand how it's diagnosed and treated in order to more effectively make decisions about your health care. And you may be finding out that getting accurate, understandable information about prostate cancer isn't all that easy, despite the multitude of information sources available in the Internet age.

Information on how to screen for, diagnose, and treat prostate cancer comes in many forms, but sometimes it's difficult to follow up on it. When a newspaper article reports promising new treatments being tested at a prominent university hospital, but there's no indication as to whether approval is imminent, how do you learn more? You see on television that the FDA has approved several new drugs for use in prostate cancer; how do you find out about them, and how do you determine which one is best? A web search of the term "prostate cancer" will bring up hundreds, if not thousands, of websites with topics ranging from scientific studies of the molecular biology of cancer, to inspirational stories about cancer survivors, to rumors, myths, and wild exaggerations about the causes of prostate cancer. How does anyone—particularly a person who never thought about cancer before and hoped he'd never have to—make sense of all this?

The information in this book is a synthesis of current medical standards, advice based on my experience as a physician, and good, old-fashioned, practical common sense. I wrote this book to help newly diagnosed patients make sense of the diagnosis and learn some of the things you can expect will happen.

Above all, I want readers to understand that you can and should ask questions, request help when you need it, and actively participate in making decisions about your treatment.

The book is divided into seven parts. Part One describes the prostate's anatomy and functions and discusses warning signs of prostate disease. Parts Two through Four describe what happens prior to treatment for prostate cancer: the risk factors, screening procedures, diagnosis, and staging of prostate cancer. Part Five discusses treatment options for prostate cancer, and Part Six describes treatment of some of the complications that arise with cancer treatment, including bone pain, incontinence, and erectile dysfunction. Part Seven addresses some of the day-to-day problems often faced by prostate cancer patients in coping with their diagnosis, treatment, and complications. An Appendix of resources is included to help readers find additional information.

The question and answer format seemed to be the most sensible way to address some of the most common questions asked by real patients. Naturally, I could not include all possible questions about prostate cancer, nor could I cover all topics as thoroughly as I would like. Thus, I've tried to present the best information available on many important topics while pointing my readers in the direction of high-quality sources of information and encouraging them to ask questions and seek assistance from their own physicians. I hope that my efforts will help some of the many men (and their families) who will confront prostate cancer in the months and years to come.

Pamela Ellsworth, MD

Preface

This book is dedicated to the men with prostate cancer, along with their families, with whom I have had the opportunity to work during the evaluation, treatment, and follow-up of their cancer throughout my residency and post-residency years. It is also dedicated to those gentlemen that I follow for prostate cancer screening. These individuals have allowed me to capture a glimpse of the magnitude of this disease and its effect on the individual and his family. All too often, we surgeons and physicians lose sight of the individual and the family in our attempts to "eradicate disease." Yet the prevalence of prostate cancer, the controversy over screening, the variety of treatment options, and the potential for treatment options to adversely affect quality of life, bring to light the need for an individual-centered approach to the treatment of prostate cancer. Choosing from the variety of treatment options, each with unique benefits and risks, as well as active surveillance and "watchful waiting" approaches, may prove overwhelming in this era of patient-driven decision making. As physicians, it is our job to educate our patients and their spouses or significant others so that they may make the most appropriate decision. Those who have shared their anger, sorrow, frustration, enthusiasm, and joy during the process of diagnosis, treatment, and follow-up have underscored the need for such extensive and personal communication. It is my hope that this book will help individuals diagnosed with or concerned about prostate cancer with some of the questions that they, their spouses, or significant others may have. I also hope that it will stimulate them to ask their physicians such questions, no matter how trivial they may perceive these questions to be.

Since writing the first four editions of this book, there have been several important changes in the evaluation and management of prostate cancer. This fifth edition will address such important changes as the development of biomarkers and their potential role in the management of prostate cancer, new prostate cancer management guidelines on clinically localized prostate cancer developed by the American Urological Association, American Society for radiation oncology and the society of urologic oncology.

I would like to thank Dr. Steven Rous for giving me the opportunity to find out how rewarding writing can be and for being a true mentor. A special thanks goes to Oliver Gill for his willingness to write about his personal experiences and to my patients with advanced prostate cancer who are willing to share their experiences. Thanks, also, to Jones & Bartlett Learning for their willingness to print a fourth edition so that patients and their families can remain "up to date" in terms of the evaluation and management of prostate cancer. Lastly, many thanks to Mary Stevens, a reader of the third edition who helped us edit the text for the third edition and improved its applicability to the layperson.

Pamela Ellsworth, MD

PART ONE

The Basics

What is the prostate gland and what does it do?

Do women have a prostate gland and PSA?

What are the signs and symptoms of an enlarged prostate (either cancer-related or benign)?

More . . .

1. What is the prostate gland and what does it do?

Gland

A structure or organ that produces substances that affect other areas of the body.

Urethra

The tube that runs from the bladder neck to the tip of the penis through which urine passes.

Posterior

The rear or back side.

The prostate gland is actually not a single gland; rather, it is composed of a collection of glands that are covered by a capsule. A **gland** is a structure or organ that produces a substance that is used in another part of the body. The prostate gland lies below the bladder, encircles the **urethra** (the tube through which one urinates), and lies in front of the rectum. Because it lies just in front of the rectum, the **posterior** (back) aspect of the prostate can be assessed during a rectal examination. The normal size of the prostate gland is about the size of a walnut (**Figure 1**, page 2).

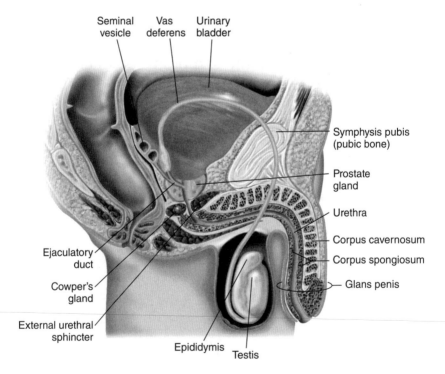

Figure 1 Anatomy of the male genitourinary system.

Data from *The Prostate Book: Sound Advice on Symptoms and Treatment*, Updated Edition by Stephen N. Rous, illustrated by Betty Goodwin. Copyright © 1992, 1988 by Stephen Rous.

The prostate gland is divided into several **zones**, or areas. These divisions are based on locations of the tissue, but they also have some significance with respect to prostate cancer. The different zones are the transition zone, the peripheral zone, and the central zone (**Figure 2**, page 3). In most prostate cancers, the tumor occurs in the peripheral zone. In a few cases, the tumor is mostly located in the transition zone, around the urethra, or toward the abdomen. In 85% of cases, the prostate cancer is **multifocal**, meaning that it is found in more than one area in the prostate. Seventy percent of prostate cancer patients with a **palpable nodule**, one that can be felt by a rectal examination, have cancer on the other side also. Another way to describe the prostate gland is to divide it into lobes. The prostate gland has five lobes:

Zones
An area of the prostate distinguished from adjacent areas.

Multifocal
Found in more than one area.

Palpable
Capable of being felt during a physical examination by an experienced doctor. In the case of prostate cancer, this refers to an abnormality of the prostate that can be felt during a rectal examination.

THE BASICS

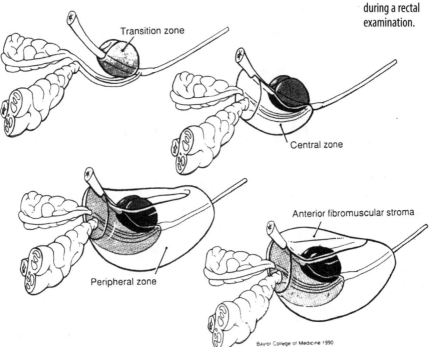

Transition zone

Central zone

Anterior fibromuscular stroma

Peripheral zone

Baylor College of Medicine 1990

Figure 2 Zones of the prostate.

Benign

A growth that is not cancerous.

two lateral lobes, a middle lobe, an anterior lobe, and a posterior lobe. **Benign** (noncancerous) enlargement of the prostate typically occurs in the lateral lobes and may also affect the middle lobe.

The prostate gland contributes substances to the ejaculate that serve as nutrients to sperm. The prostate gland has a high amount of zinc in it. The reason for this is not clear, but it appears to help in fighting off infections.

2. Do women have a prostate gland and PSA?

No, women do not have prostate glands. However, small amounts of a chemical typically produced by the prostate, **prostate-specific antigen** (**PSA**), are found in certain tissues and fluids in women, including normal breast tissue, breast fluid, breast cancer tissue, and other female tumors.

Prostate-specific antigen (PSA)

A chemical produced by benign and cancerous prostate tissue. The level tends to be higher with prostate cancer.

3. What are the signs and symptoms of an enlarged prostate (either cancer-related or benign)?

The prostate gland in the adult male is normally about 20 to 25 cc in size. Over time, the prostate gland may grow as a result of benign enlargement of the prostate, known as **benign prostatic hyperplasia** (**BPH**), or as a result of prostate cancer. Enlargement of the prostate gland may cause changes in urinary symptoms; however, the severity of urinary symptoms does not correlate with the size of the prostate. In fact, some men with mildly enlarged prostates (for example, 40 cc) may be more symptomatic than men with greatly enlarged (> 100 cc)

Benign prostatic hyperplasia (BPH)

Noncancerous enlargement of the prostate.

prostate glands. The symptoms of an enlarged prostate are caused by the prostate's resistance to the outflow of urine and the bladder's response to this resistance. Common symptoms include:

- Getting up at night to urinate one or more times per night (**nocturia**)
- Urinating more frequently than every two hours during the daytime
- Feeling that you have to urinate, but when you attempt to, finding that it takes a while for the urine to come out (**hesitancy**)
- Straining or pushing to get your urine stream started and/or to maintain your stream
- Dribbling urine near the completion of voiding
- A urine stream that stops and starts during voiding (**intermittency**)
- Feeling of incomplete emptying after voiding such that you feel that you could void again shortly

4. What is PSA? What is the normal PSA value?

PSA stands for prostate-specific antigen. PSA is a chemical that is produced by prostate cells, both normal and cancerous. PSA is not produced significantly by other cells in the body, however, it is produced by salivary gland tissue in low concentration. Normally, only a small amount of PSA gets into the bloodstream. However, when the prostate is irritated, inflamed, or damaged, such as in prostatitis and prostate cancer, PSA leaks into the bloodstream more easily, causing the level of PSA in the blood to be higher. The normal range is usually 0 to 4 ng/mL; however, in younger men, a lower range is used. The normal range for PSA varies with

THE BASICS

Nocturia
Awakening at night with the desire to void.

Hesitancy
A delay in the start of the urine stream during voiding.

Intermittency
An inability to complete voiding and empty the bladder with one single contraction of the bladder. A stopping and starting of the urine stream during urination.

age and race. There is an online prostate cancer risk calculator that can be used to help determine your risk of prostate cancer, www.prostatecancer-riskcalculator.com.

Once a baseline normal PSA has been obtained, the actual number becomes less important, and the rate of change of the PSA over time becomes more important.

5. What is free : total PSA?

Bound PSA

PSA attached to the proteins in the bloodstream.

Free PSA

The PSA present that is not bound to proteins. It is often expressed as a ratio of free PSA to total PSA in terms of percent, which is the free PSA divided by the total PSA × 100.

PSA is found in two forms in the bloodstream: PSA that is attached to chemicals (proteins) is **bound PSA**, and PSA that is not attached to proteins is called **free PSA**. The amount of each form is measured, and a ratio of the free PSA to the free plus bound (or total) PSA is calculated. The higher this number, the less likely that prostate cancer is present. A free PSA value greater than 14–25% suggests that the presence of prostate cancer is less likely. This ratio may be helpful in individuals with mildly elevated PSAs in the 4–10 ng/mL range for whom the doctor is deciding whether to perform a prostate biopsy.

6. What causes the PSA to rise?

Anything that irritates or inflames the prostate can increase the PSA, such as a urinary tract infection, prostate stones, a recent urinary catheter or cystoscopy (a look into the bladder through a specialized telescope-like instrument), recent prostate biopsy, or prostate surgery. Sexual intercourse may increase the PSA up to 10%, and a vigorous rectal examination or prostatic massage before the PSA blood test is drawn may also increase the PSA. Benign enlargement of the prostate may also increase the PSA because more prostate cells

are present, thus more PSA is produced. Benign prostatic hyperplasia (BPH) tends to produce less PSA than
prostate cancer, so with BPH the PSA density (the
amount of PSA/volume of prostate) is lower than with
prostate cancer. Because the prostate gland can continue
to grow as one ages, the PSA may increase slightly from
year to year, reflecting this growth. Some argue that
the PSA should not change by more than 0.7 ng/mL
per year or by 20% of the previous level if the increase is
secondary to benign growth of the prostate. There are
studies that suggest that long-term PSA velocity may
help differentiate clinically insignificant prostate cancer
from life-threatening prostate cancer (*Rev Urol* 2013;
15(4): 204–206). The rate of change in the PSA over a
period of time is called the **PSA velocity**.

PSA velocity
The rate of
change in PSA
over time.

7. Are there medications that may affect the PSA? Does testosterone therapy cause the PSA to increase?

Yes, some medications can affect the PSA. Finasteride
(Proscar), dutasteride (Avodart), and a combination of
dutasteride and tamsulosin (Jalyn), medications used to
shrink the prostate in men with benign enlargement of
the prostate, decreases the PSA up to 50%. No matter
what your initial PSA is this decrease in PSA predictably
occurs. Any sustained increases in PSA while you are
taking Proscar or Avodart (provided that you are taking
the Proscar regularly) should be evaluated. The percentage of free PSA (the amount of free PSA divided by the
amount of total PSA) is not significantly decreased by
Proscar or Avodart and should remain stable while you
are taking Proscar or Avodart. Other medications that
can decrease the amount of testosterone produced by
your testicles, such as ketoconazole, may decrease the

PSA. Decreasing the amount of testosterone may cause both benign and cancerous prostate tissue to shrink. Testosterone is broken down in the body to a chemical, dihydrotestosterone, which is responsible for the stimulation of prostate growth. Thus, the addition of testosterone may stimulate the growth of normal prostate cells and possibly prostate cancer cells. Because normal prostate cells produce PSA, it is not unreasonable to expect that an increase in the normal cells present in the prostate would lead to an increase in the PSA. Prostate cancer is composed of both hormone-sensitive and hormone-insensitive cells. The hormone-insensitive cells grow regardless of the availability of testosterone or its breakdown products, whereas the hormone-sensitive cells appear to be dependent on the male hormone for growth. Thus, the addition of testosterone may affect the growth of these hormone-sensitive cells. Testosterone therapy has not been shown to cause the development of prostate cancer.

Testosterone replacement therapy (TRT)

The practice of giving testosterone to treat conditions in which the testes do not produce enough testosterone.

Several studies have assessed the effect of **testosterone replacement therapy** (**TRT**) on PSA level; on average men on TRT will have an associated increase in PSA of 0.30 ng/mL/yr, with older men having an increase of 0.43 ng/mL/yr (Bhasin S, Singh AB, et al. Managing the risks of prostate disease during testosterone replacement therapy in older men: recommendations for a standardized monitoring plan, *J Androl.* 2003; 24: 299–311).

8. Is there anything special that I should do if I am on testosterone therapy?

Because there is theoretical risk that testosterone therapy can cause an undetected prostate cancer to grow, you should have a digital rectal examination (DRE) and get a PSA level more regularly, within 3 months of starting testosterone therapy and then in accordance with guidelines for prostate cancer screening. If there is a significant increase in your PSA or a change in your rectal examination while you are on testosterone therapy, the testosterone should be discontinued and a transrectal ultrasound (TRUS)–guided prostate biopsy should be performed. Some clinicians recommend performing a prostate biopsy on any patient on testosterone replacement therapy with a yearly PSA increase of 1.0 ng/mL or more. If the PSA increases by 0.7 to 0.9 ng/mL in 1 year, repeat the PSA in 3–6 months and perform a biopsy if there is any further increase.

9. Can I have my PSA done anywhere?

It is best to have your PSA obtained at the same lab each time because different labs may use different forms of PSA testing. The PSA Hybritech Tandem-R PSA test can detect PSA at a level of 0.1 ng/mL, whereas some of the newer PSA tests, such as the Abbott IMx, Yang Proscheck, and Diagnostic Products Immulite, can detect PSA at levels of 0.01–0.04 ng/mL. To minimize lab variability and to avoid unnecessary anxiety, repeat blood tests, or biopsy, it is best to have your PSA performed by the same lab each year.

10. Are there any other markers for prostate cancer?

There are a number of blood- (serum) and urine-based **biomarkers** that may be helpful for the detection as well as management of prostate cancer (see **Table 1**, page 10). Although many of these tests are "approved" by regulatory agencies, they may still be considered investigational/

Biomarker

A characteristic that is objectively measured and evaluated as an indicator of normal biological processes, pathologic processes or pharmacological responses to a therapeutic intervention.

Table 1 Biomarkers of Prostate Cancer

Biomarker	Prior to Initial Biopsy	Negative Prior Biopsy/ Re-biopsy	Positive Biopsy Risk Stratification	Follow Up After Surgery/ EBRT/ Brachytherapy
PCA3		•		
TMPRSS2-ERG		•		
ExoDx Prostate Intelliscore		•		
SCHLAP1		•	•	
Select MDx	•	•		
Confirm MDx		•		
4Kscore	•			
PHI	•			
Prostarix	•	•		
OncotypeDx			•	
Prolaris			•	•
ELAVL1			•	
Decipher			•	•

experimental and not medically necessary by some insurance companies. Current National Comprehensive Cancer Network guidelines indicate that biomarkers may be helpful in select patients.

PCA3 (prostate cancer gene 3) is over expressed in prostate cancer cells. Its product can be measured in urine specimens obtained after DRE. The sensitivity and specificity of PCA3 vary considerably depending on the cutoff used: a cutoff of 25 is suggested for a recently approved PCA3 assay. PCA3 is approved for use in men 50 years of age or older who have had one or more previous negative biopsies, but didn't have a finding of atypical small acinar cells in the most recent biopsy.

The University of Michigan Mlabs offers the new test, Mi-Prostate (MiPS), which incorporates blood PSA levels and two molecular markers specific for prostate cancer in one final score. The two urine markers are related to RNA from the PCA3 gene that is overactive in 95% of prostate cancers and the second marker is RNA that is made when 2 genes (**TMPRSS2** and **ERG**) abnormally fuse. The presence of this fusion RNA in a man's urine is ultra-specific for prostate cancer.

ExoDx Prostate Intelliscore urine exosome assay is a urine test that detects 3 important genetic biomarkers to help determine the risk of Gleason 6 and 7 prostate cancer (see Question 38) and benign (noncancerous) disease on the initial prostate biopsy. The 3 genes measured in the urine are ERG, PCA3, and SPDEF.

Prostate Health Index (PHI) is a mathematical formula that combines the levels of 3 different forms of PSA (prostate specific antigen)—total PSA, free PSA, and (–2)proPSA to help predict the likelihood of finding prostate cancer in the biopsy tissue. Higher PHI values have been shown to be associated with more aggressive prostate cancers.

The **4K score** test is a blood test. This test measures blood levels of 4 proteins—total PSA, free PSA, intact PSA, and human kallikrein 2. These values are combined with the individual's age, presence or absence of a nodule in the prostate during a DRE, and prior biopsy (yes or no). This information is fit into an algorithm to calculate the risk of having Gleason 7 or higher prostate cancer (see Question 38).

THE BASICS

TMPRSS2-ERG

A prostate specific gene which is an **oncogene** for prostate cancer.

Oncogene

A gene that in certain situations can turn a cell into a cancer cell.

ExoDx prostate intelliscore urine exosome assay

Score based on 3 genes (ERG, PCA 3, SPDEF)—helps determine risk of Gleason 6, 7, and benign disease on initial prostate biopsy.

Prostate health index (PHI)

A mathematical formula that relies on differing proportions of specific biomarkers—can be helpful in distinguishing between benign prostatic hypertrophy (BPH) and prostate cancer.

4K score

Determined by levels of total PSA, free PSA, intact PSA, and human kallikrein 2—helps improve diagnostic accuracy for clinically significant prostate cancer.

Confirm MDx

Special gene test that uses DNA methylation to detect likelihood of prostate cancer on a repeat biopsy.

Confirm MDx is a tissue-based test that uses prostate tissue obtained from a prior negative biopsy. It measures 3 genes: GSTP1, APC, and RASSF1. This test helps predict the likelihood of detection of prostate cancer on repeat prostate biopsy.

Select MDx

Urinary 2 gene assay (HOX 6 and DLK1) used to identify high grade prostate cancer.

Select MDx is a urine-based test. It measures 2 genes (HOXC6 and DLX1). It is currently being used in individuals being considered for a prostate biopsy or who have had a negative prostate biopsy but have high risk factors for prostate cancer such as an abnormal prostate on a DRE, family history of prostate cancer, or a high PSA level.

Prostarix is a gene-based urine test that helps in decision-making regarding initial or repeat biopsies in men with a negative DRE and an elevated PSA level.

IsoPSA

A new test that is based on the fact that molecules (proteins) produced by cancer cells have different 3D structures than the same proteins produced by normal cells.

Investigators are evaluating a new PSA test, **IsoPSA**, that is based on the fact that chemicals produced by cancer cells have different 3D structures (isoforms). One study using IsoPSA allowed the investigator to distinguish between more aggressive prostate cancer and less aggressive cancer. This is new and requires further research.

PART TWO

Prostate Cancer

What is prostate cancer?

How common is prostate cancer?

What are the risk factors for prostate cancer,
and who is at risk?

More . . .

11. What is prostate cancer?

Cell

The smallest unit of the body. Tissues in the body are made up of cells.

Tumor

Abnormal tissue growth that may be cancerous or noncancerous (benign).

Cancer

Abnormal and uncontrolled growth of cells in the body that may spread, injure areas of the body, and/or lead to death.

Malignancy

Uncontrolled growth of cells that can spread to other areas of the body and cause death.

Lymph

A clear fluid that is found throughout the body. Lymph fluid helps fight infections.

Lymph node(s)

Small, bean-shaped glands that are found throughout the body. Lymph fluid passes through the lymph nodes, which filter out bacteria, cancer cells, and toxic chemicals.

Prostate cancer is a malignant growth of the glandular cells of the prostate. Our body is composed of billions of **cells**; they are the smallest unit in the body. Normally, each cell functions for a while, then dies and is replaced in an organized manner. This results in the appropriate number of cells being present to carry out necessary cell functions. Sometimes there can be an uncontrolled replacement of cells, leaving the cells unable to organize as they did before. Such abnormal growth of cells is called a **tumor**. Tumors may be benign (noncancerous) or malignant (cancerous). **Cancer** is abnormal cell growth and disorder such that the "cancer cells" can grow without the normal controls and limits. A **malignancy** is a cancerous growth that has the potential to spread and cause damage to other tissues of the body or even lead to death. Cancers can spread locally into surrounding tissues, or cancer cells can break away from the tumor and enter body fluids, such as the blood and lymph, and spread to other parts of the body. **Lymph** is an almost clear fluid that drains waste from cells. This fluid travels in vessels to the **lymph nodes**, small, bean-shaped structures that filter unwanted substances, such as cancer cells and bacteria, out of the fluid. Lymph nodes may become filled with cancer cells.

As with most cancers, prostate cancer is not contagious.

12. How common is prostate cancer?

There are more than 100 different types of cancer. In the United States, a man has a 50% chance of developing some type of cancer in his lifetime. In American men, excluding skin cancer, prostate cancer is the most common cancer. It is estimated that 161,360 new cases of prostate cancer will occur in the United States in 2017 (**Table 2**, page 15). Rates of prostate cancer in African Americans is significantly higher.

Prostate cancer is the third leading cause of cancer death in men. It is estimated that there will be 26,730 deaths in 2017. Prostate cancer death rates have been decreasing since the 1990s with death rates decreasing more rapidly in African Americans than in Caucasian males (**Table 3**, page 16).

13. What are the risk factors for prostate cancer, and who is at risk? Is there anything that decreases the risk of developing prostate cancer?

Theoretically, all men are at risk for developing prostate cancer. There are several risk factors for prostate cancer, some are modifiable (you can change them) and others are not modifiable (see **Table 4**, page 17). The prevalence of prostate cancer increases with age, and the increase with age is greater for prostate cancer than for any other cancer.

Table 2 Cancer Statistics for Men in the United States, 2017

Cancer Site	Estimated Number of New Cases
Prostate	161,360
Lung and bronchus	116,990
Colon and rectum	71,420

Data from 2017 American Cancer Society, Inc. Surveillance Research. Cancer Facts and Figures. www.cancer.org/acs.

Table 3 2017 Estimated New Cases and Deaths for Men — Top Five

Location	% of All Cancer Cases	Deaths	% of All Cancer Cases
Prostate	19%	Lung and bronchus	27%
Lung and bronchus	14%	Colon and rectum	9%
Colon and rectum	9%	Prostate	8%
Bladder	7%	Pancreas	7%
Melanoma of skin	5%	Liver and intrahepatic bile duct	6%

Data from 2017 American Cancer Society, Inc. Surveillance Research. Cancer Facts and Figures. www.cancer.org/acs

Basically, every ten years after the age of 40, the incidence of prostate cancer nearly doubles, with a risk of 10% for men in their 50s increasing to 70% for those in their 80s. However, in most older men, the prostate cancer does not grow quickly enough to cause problems; many die of other causes and are not identified as having prostate cancer before their death.

Prostate cancer is 66% more common among African Americans, and it is twice as likely to be fatal in African Americans as in Caucasians. However, blacks in Africa have one of the lowest rates of prostate cancer in the world. Males of Asian descent living in the United States have lower rates of prostate cancer than Caucasians, but higher rates than Asian males in their native countries. Japan appears to have the lowest prostate cancer death rate, compared with Switzerland, which has the highest.

Prostate cancer is related to sex hormones. Prostate cancer rarely develops in men who had their testicles removed (**castration**) at an early age. There is a correlation between prostate cancer and high levels of testosterone. There does not appear to be any clear correlation between body size and risk of prostate cancer;

Castration

The removal of both testicles.

Table 4 Risk Factors for Prostate Cancer

Modifiable	Non-modifiable
Diet	Genetics
Exercise	Age
Exposures (radiation—ionizing and UV [sun])	Sex
	Ethnicity
Smoking	
Obesity	

however, men with prostate cancer who had weight gain in early adulthood tend to have more aggressive cancers. Smoking is associated with a moderate increased risk of prostate cancer, particularly heavy smokers. Physical activity appears to decrease the risk of prostate cancer.

The effects of a vasectomy on the risk of prostate cancer are unclear. Some studies have demonstrated an increased risk of prostate cancer with a vasectomy, but these individuals tended to have a lower-grade, lower-stage prostate cancer that is associated with a better prognosis. Other studies have failed to confirm an increased risk of prostate cancer after a vasectomy. **Vasectomy** is the minor surgical sterilization procedure in which the **vas deferens** (the sperm duct) is cut and either clipped, tied, or cauterized to prevent it from reattaching itself. A vasectomy does not affect testosterone production or the release of testosterone from the testicles into the bloodstream; it only prevents sperm from leaving the testis. Current medical wisdom holds that a vasectomy does not increase your risk of prostate cancer.

There appears to be an increased risk of prostate cancer in veterans exposed to **Agent Orange** and in individuals exposed to ionizing radiation, and ultraviolet radiation from the sun may increase prostate cancer risk.

Vasectomy

A procedure in which the vas deferens are cut and tied off, clipped, or cauterized to prevent the exit of sperm from the testicles. It makes a man sterile.

Vas deferens

A tiny tube that connects the testicles to the urethra through which sperm passes.

Agent Orange

A herbicide containing trace amounts of a toxic chemical dioxin that was used during the Vietnam War to defoliate areas of the forest.

Dietary (see Question 17) and genetic (hereditary) factors (see Question 16) may also play a role in the risk of developing cancer.

The Cancer Risk Calculator for Prostate Cancer has been developed as a tool to help identify one's risk of having prostate cancer. The calculator may be applied to men age 50 years or older, with no previous diagnosis of prostate cancer and DRE and PSA results less than 1 year old. The calculator may also be applied to men undergoing a prostate cancer screening with PSA and DRE, as it was developed from the Prostate Cancer Prevention Trial. The calculator is designed to provide a preliminary assessment of risk of prostate cancer if a prostate biopsy is performed. One can find the prostate cancer risk calculator online, either by Googling "cancer risk calculator for prostate cancer" or by going to the National Cancer Institute website and looking under early detection research network.

A recent study called the Prostate Cancer Prevention Trial (PCPT) demonstrated that finasteride (Proscar) at a dose of 5 mg/day decreases the likelihood of developing prostate cancer by 25% when compared to a placebo (candy pill). In addition, finasteride decreased the risk of high-grade prostatic intraepithelial neoplasia (PIN) (which may be a precursor of prostate cancer) by about the same rate. Side effects of finasteride include decreased sexual desire, impotence, and decreased ejaculate volume (www.cancer.gov/cancertopics/factsheet/pcptqa).

Results of the Reduction by Dutasteride of Prostate Cancer (REDUCE) trial showed that the 5-alpha-reductase inhibitor dutasteride at doses of 0.5 mg a day decreased the relative risk of prostate cancer by 23% compared to placebo. Furthermore, the risk was markedly decreased in the number of high-grade tumors, with no absolute increase in incidence compared to a placebo.

Asymptomatic men with a PSA less than or equal to 3.0 ng/mL who are regularly screened with PSA or who are anticipating undergoing an annual PSA screening for the early detection of prostate cancer may benefit from a discussion of both of the benefits of 5-alpha-reductase inhibitors for 7 years for the prevention of prostate cancer and the potential risks (2–4% increase in reported erectile dysfunction and gynecomastia [enlarged and/or painful breasts] and decrease in ejaculate volume in those receiving finasteride in the study compared to those receiving the placebo).

Obesity is associated with an increased risk of prostate cancer. Some studies have demonstrated that obesity is associated with a greater risk of more advanced prostate cancer and of dying from prostate cancer.

Inflammation/infection of the prostate does not appear to increase the risk of prostate cancer.

14. I have a family member with prostate cancer. Am I at risk?

In certain cases, it appears that the risk for prostate cancer is passed on to males in the family. The younger the family member is when he is diagnosed with prostate cancer, the higher the risk is for male relatives to have prostate cancer at a younger age. The risk also increases with the number of relatives affected with prostate cancer. The risk appears to be higher in men under 65 years of age compared to older men and if the affected relative was a brother rather than a father.

15. I have sons. Are they at risk for prostate cancer? And, if so, at what age should they start screening?

Yes, there is an increased risk for all male relatives, including brothers, sons, cousins, and nephews. Your sons' risk varies with your age at detection. The younger you are at diagnosis, the higher the risk for your sons. If your age is 72 or older at the time of diagnosis of prostate cancer, then your sons' risk is probably no greater than that of the general population.

Screening of your sons should begin at age 40, and a DRE should be performed and a PSA obtained, both of which should be repeated yearly thereafter.

Screening of your sons should begin at age 40, and a DRE should be performed and a PSA obtained, both of which should be repeated yearly thereafter. It may also be helpful for your sons to make some preventive dietary and lifestyle changes now (see Question 17).

16. Are there genes that put people at risk for prostate cancer?

It is thought that 9% of all prostate cancers, and more than 40% of prostate cancers occurring in younger males, are related to genetic causes. Abnormalities of genes of chromosome 1 and the X chromosome are associated with an increased risk of prostate cancer. One such gene, the HPC1 gene, appears to cause about one-third of all inherited cases of prostate cancer. There also appears to be a gene that is carried on the X chromosome (the chromosome passed on to the male by his mother) that may increase the risk of prostate cancer. This X chromosome–related increased risk of prostate cancer might somehow play a part in the identification of a higher incidence of prostate cancer in male relatives of women with breast cancer.

Single-**nucleotide** polymorphisms (SNPs) in five chromosomal regions—three at 8q24 and one each at 17q12 and 17q24.3—have been associated with prostate cancer.

Changes in the **BRCA1** and BRCA2 genes may increase prostate cancer risk in men and are associated with an increased risk of breast and ovarian cancer in women.

There is a test called the "color test" (Genome dx) that allows an individual with prostate cancer to determine if there is a hereditary (genetic) component to his prostate cancer. It also assesses the risk for other common cancers. The test analyzes 30 genes. This test may be performed using saliva or blood.

17. How does diet affect my risk of prostate cancer?

No diet study has proven that diet and nutrition can directly cause or prevent prostate cancer. However, many studies that look at dietary intake and cancer suggest that there may be an association.

Men who eat a lot of red meat or high-fat dairy products appear to have a slightly higher risk of prostate cancer. They tend to eat fewer fruits and vegetables. It is unclear if the increase in risk is related to an increase in red meat consumption or high-fat dairy products or the decrease in fruits/vegetables.

Increased calcium intake may lead to an increased risk of prostate cancer; similarly, dairy foods may increase risk of prostate cancer. There has not been a demonstrated risk with normal calcium intake.

Nucleotide

Any of the various compounds consisting of a nucleoside combined with a phosphate group and forming the basic constituents of DNA and RNA.

BRCA1

Gene which may increase the risk of prostate cancer.

The data regarding an association with serum levels of vitamin D and prostate cancer are conflicting. Dietary intake of vitamin D does not appear to be protective against prostate cancer; however, one study did show a 40% risk reduction in men taking > 600 IU of supplemental vitamin D, compared to those not taking vitamin D supplements. High levels of fructose, a form of sugar, may be associated with a lower risk of prostate cancer. Lycopene, a carotenoid (chemicals that give orange, red, or yellow coloring to plants) has been shown in some studies to decrease the risk of prostate cancer. Lycopene is found in high levels in tomatoes and is beneficial only if one eats cooked tomatoes, such as tomato sauce, not tomato juice. Further studies are needed to determine the true impact of such dietary factors on prostate cancer risk.

Selenium and vitamin E were thought to potentially decrease prostate cancer risk. However, a clinical trial of > 35,000 men, the Selenium and Vitamin E Cancer Prevention Trial (SELECT), found that selenium and vitamin E supplements, taken alone or together, for an average of 5 years did not prevent prostate cancer and may even be harmful to some men.

18. Do African Americans have a higher risk of prostate cancer?

African–American men are more likely to get prostate cancer at a younger age, and they often have a more aggressive cancer.

African-American men are more likely to get prostate cancer at a younger age, and they often have a more aggressive cancer. Of all population groups in the world, African-American men have the highest rate of prostate cancer. The reason for this is not known. Because they are at higher risk, African-American men should start prostate cancer screening at a younger age than Caucasian men (see Question 28).

19. What are the warning signs of prostate cancer?

Prostate cancer gives no typical warning signs that it is present in your body. It often grows very slowly, and some of the symptoms related to the enlargement of the prostate are typical of noncancerous enlargement of the prostate, known as benign prostatic hyperplasia (BPH).

With more advanced disease, you may have fatigue, weight loss, and generalized aches and pains.

When the disease has spread to the bones, it may cause pain in the area. Bone pain may present in different ways. In some men, it may cause continuous pain, while in others, the pain may be intermittent. It may be confined to a particular area of the body or move around the body; it may be variable during the day and respond differently to rest and activity. If there is significant weakening of the bone(s), fractures (breaks in the bone) may occur. More common sites of bone metastases include the hips, back, ribs, and shoulders. Some of these sites are also common locations for arthritis, so the presence of pain in any of these areas is not definitive for prostate cancer.

If prostate cancer spreads locally to the lymph nodes, it often does not cause any symptoms. Rarely, if there is extensive lymph node involvement, leg swelling may occur.

In patients with advanced cancer that has spread to the spine, paralysis can occur if the nerves are compressed because of either the collapse of the spine or a tumor growing into the spine.

If the prostate cancer grows into the floor (bottom) of the bladder, or if a large amount of cancer is present in the pelvic lymph nodes, one or both **ureters** (the tubes

Ureters

Tubes that connect the kidneys to the bladder, through which urine passes into the bladder.

23

that drain urine from the kidneys into the bladder) can be obstructed. Signs and symptoms of ureteral obstruction include decreased urine volume, no urine volume if both ureters are blocked, back pain, nausea, vomiting, and possibly fevers if infections occur.

Blood in the urine and blood in the ejaculate are usually not related to prostate cancer; however, if these are present, you should seek urologic evaluation.

In individuals with widespread metastatic disease, bleeding problems can occur. In addition, patients with prostate cancer may develop anemia. The anemia may be related to extensive tumor in the bone, hormonal therapy, or the length of time you have had the cancer. Because the blood count tends to drop slowly, you may not have any symptoms of anemia. Some individuals with very significant anemia may have weakness, orthostatic hypotension (lowering of the blood pressure when you stand up), dizziness, shortness of breath, and the feeling of being ill and tired.

20. What causes prostate cancer?

The exact causes of prostate cancer are not known. Prostate cancer may develop because of changes in genes. Alterations in androgen (male hormone) related genes have been associated with an increased risk of cancer. Alterations in genes may be caused by environmental factors, such as diet. The more abnormal the gene, the higher is the likelihood of developing prostate cancer. In rare cases, prostate cancer may be inherited. In such cases, 88% of the individuals will have prostate cancer by the age of 85 years. Males who have a particular gene, the breast cancer mutation (BRCA1), have a threefold higher risk of developing prostate cancer than do other men. Changes in a certain chromosome, p53, in prostate cancer are associated with high-grade, aggressive prostate cancer.

21. What causes prostate cancer to grow?

Prostate cancer, similar to breast cancer, is hormone sensitive. Prostate cancer growth is stimulated by the male hormones testosterone and dihydrotestosterone (a chemical that the body makes from testosterone). Testosterone is responsible for many normal changes, both physical and behavioral, that occur in a man's life, such as voice change and hair growth. The testis makes almost 90% of the testosterone in the body. A small amount of testosterone is made by the **adrenal glands** (a paired set of glands found above the kidneys that produce a variety of substances and hormones that are essential for daily living). In the bones, a chemical called transferrin, which is made by the liver and stored in the bones, also appears to stimulate the growth of prostate cancer cells. When cancers develop, they secrete chemicals that cause blood vessels to grow into the cancer and bring nutrients to the cancer so that it can grow.

Adrenal glands

Glands located above each kidney. These glands produce several different hormones, including sex hormones.

22. Where does prostate cancer spread?

As the prostate cancer grows, it grows through the prostate, the prostate capsule, and the fat that surrounds the prostate capsule. Because the prostate gland lies below the bladder and attaches to it, the prostate cancer can also grow up into the base of the bladder.

Prostate cancer can also grow into the **seminal vesicles** (paired structures that produce fluid that is part of the ejaculate volume), which are located adjacent to the

Seminal vesicles

Glandular structures that are located above and behind the prostate. They produce fluid that is part of the ejaculate.

prostate. It may continue to grow locally in the pelvis into muscles within the pelvis; into the rectum, which lies behind the prostate; or into the sidewall of the pelvis. The spread of cancer to other sites is called metastasis. When prostate cancer spreads outside of the capsule and the fatty tissue, it usually goes to two main areas in the body: the lymph nodes that drain the prostate and the bones. The more commonly involved lymph nodes are those in the pelvis (**Figure 3**, page 27), and bones that are more commonly affected are the spine (backbones) and the ribs. Less commonly, prostate cancer can spread to solid organs in the body, such as the liver.

23. Does having a prior transurethral prostatectomy without detection of any cancer protect or assure me that I don't have and won't develop prostate cancer?

Transurethral prostatectomy (TURP)

A surgical technique performed under anesthesia using a specialized instrument similar to the cystoscope that allows the surgeon to remove the prostatic tissue that is bulging into the urethra and blocking the flow of urine through the urethra. After a TURP, the outer rim of the prostate remains.

The answer to this question is no for several reasons. Remember, prostate cancer tends to develop in the peripheral zone of the prostate, whereas benign growth of the prostate (BPH) tends to occur in the transition zone. The goal of the **transurethral prostatectomy** (**TURP**) is to remove all of the obstructing prostatic tissue; thus, the transition zone tissue is resected, and depending on the skill and thoroughness of your urologist, variable amounts of the peripheral zone tissue are also resected. However, TURP does not remove all of your prostate tissue. At the completion of a TURP, you are still left with the remaining prostate tissue and thus need to continue with prostate cancer screening. The

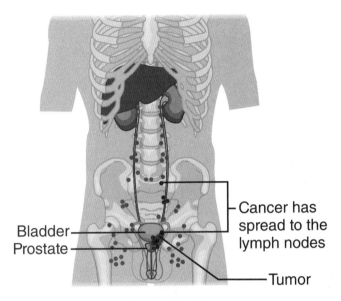

Bladder
Prostate

Cancer has
spread to the
lymph nodes

Tumor

Figure 3 Lymph node drainage from the prostate.

only surgical procedure that removes all prostate tissue is a radical prostatectomy. Some men with very large prostates undergo an open prostatectomy for benign enlargement of the prostate. This procedure does not remove all of the prostate tissue either; however, it tends to remove more than a TURP.

Remember that you are not born with prostate cancer. Prostate cancer develops over time, and the incidence increases with age. Thus, if you had your TURP at a younger age, there is still a chance that as you age, a prostate cancer will develop, and you should participate in prostate cancer screening if this is appropriate for you.

PART THREE

Evaluation for Prostate Cancer

How do you detect prostate cancer?

What is prostate cancer screening?

Will my insurance cover prostate cancer screening and treatment?

More . . .

24. How do you detect prostate cancer?

Prostate cancer often does not cause any signs or symptoms, and there are no signs or symptoms specific to prostate cancer. In the earlier stages, it may not cause any perceptible changes in your overall health that will make you aware of the cancer's presence. Currently, a high PSA is the most common indication for prostate biopsy. However, prostate cancer may occur in men with a normal PSA, and this is why the rectal examination is important. Even if you have a normal PSA, you should undergo a prostate biopsy if a rectal examination reveals a firm or nodular area. A combination of PSA and a DRE is the best screening for prostate cancer. Occasionally, prostate cancer is detected when the pathologist examines prostate tissue that was removed during a TURP or open prostatectomy for BPH. This occurs in about 10–15% of individuals with prostate cancer. If prostate cancer is not detected early and is identified in the later stages, it may be detected as part of a workup for bone pain, urinary tract obstruction, weight loss, or hematuria.

Biomarkers, including PHI, 4K score, PCA3, and MiPS, may be helpful in assessing the risk for prostate cancer (see Table 1, page 10).

25. What is prostate cancer screening?

A combination of PSA and a DRE is the best screening for prostate cancer.

The goal of any "screening" is to evaluate populations of people in an effort to diagnose the disease early. Thus, the goal of prostate cancer screening is the early detection of prostate cancer, ideally at the "curable" stage. Prostate cancer screening includes both a DRE and a serum PSA. Each of these is important in the screening process, and an abnormality in either warrants further evaluation. Only about 25% (one quarter) of prostate cancers are revealed by rectal examination; most are detected by an abnormal PSA. Some studies suggest that even with PSA-based prostate cancer screening, up to 15% of men will have undetected prostate cancer. PCA3 is a newer screening tool for the detection of prostate cancer (see Question 10). PCA3 is a new urine-based screening tool that is FDA approved for the detection of prostate cancer (see Question 9). PHI is a biomarker that is associated with prostate cancer. Both PCA3 and PHI may be helpful in determining the need for prostate biopsy (see Table 1, page 10).

In 2012 the U.S. Preventive Services Task Force recommendation on PSA screening concluded that the potential benefits do not outweigh the harms. However, more recently the new Task Force has changed its collective mind and new draft guidelines leave the decision about prostate cancer screening to individual men in consultation with their doctors. The Task Force does not recommend screening in men 70 years of age and older. The American Urological Association (AUA) issued new guidelines for PSA screening in May 2013 and noted:

- PSA screening in men 40 years of age is not recommended.
- Routine screening in men between the ages of 40 to 54 years at average risk for prostate cancer is not recommended.
- For men ages 55 to 69 years, the decision to undergo PSA screening involves weighing the benefits of preventing prostate cancer mortality in 1 man for every 1000 men screened over a decade against the known potential harms associated with screening and treatment. Hence, the recommendation is for shared decision-making.

- To reduce the harms of screening, a routine screening interval of every 2 years or more may be preferred over annual screening in those men who have participated in shared decision-making and decided on screening. It is thought that screening intervals of 2 years preserve the majority of benefits and reduce overdiagnosis and false positives.

- Routine PSA screening is not recommended for men > 70 years of age or any male with < 10- to 15-year life expectancy.

26. Will my insurance cover prostate cancer screening and treatment?

At this point, Medicare covers an annual DRE and PSA for qualified Medicare patients age 50 and older. Most health insurance providers are also providing similar coverage. The costs of the various treatments for prostate cancer vary from institution to institution. Most HMOs cover treatment of prostate cancer if the treatment is performed by an HMO-affiliated physician. If you receive care outside of the HMO system, then you may be responsible for the cost of your treatment. If you have questions regarding insurance coverage, it is always best to check with your insurance company before you start screening and treatment to make sure that you are fully aware of your coverage and its possible limitations. Medicare Part B covers a DRE once every 12 months, and PSA once every 12 months. Individualized state mandates for prostate cancer screening exist.

Insurance coverage for the use of biomarkers in the evaluation of men suspected of having prostate cancer and for guiding treatment of prostate cancer may vary. Thus, it may be helpful to check with your insurance company prior to obtaining the test.

27. Why do some primary care providers discourage or not discuss prostate cancer screening?

The PSA test is a sensitive, but not specific, test for prostate cancer, but elevated PSA can stem from circumstances other than cancer, as noted in Questions 6 and 7. This means that a fair number of men who undergo TRUS-guided prostate biopsies for an elevated PSA do not have prostate cancer, and their worries about cancer are unnecessary. In addition, many argue that with PSA testing, we may be detecting a large number of "clinically **occult**" prostate cancers (cancers that would have gone undetected if not for the PSA test) that would not have caused the individual any harm. Identification and subsequent treatment of such cancers may place the individual at unnecessary risk for erectile dysfunction and urinary troubles including incontinence. Indeed, detection of occult, non–life-threatening cancers was believed to be the reason for the large number of prostate cancers detected when PSA testing was first used; however, the numbers have decreased, suggesting that this is not entirely the case. Until recently, it was argued that the early detection of prostate cancer did not affect survival; however, recent long-term studies have shown a positive impact of prostate cancer screening on prostate cancer-related survival. The identification of several new biomarkers may help in the identification of men with clinically significant prostate cancer who warrant treatment as well as those at risk for disease progression (see Question 47). Prostate cancer screening is not mandatory; it is your choice whether to have it. You should discuss the pros and cons of prostate cancer screening with your primary care provider and consider how it relates to your overall medical health as you make your decision. If you wish to have a PSA test and your primary

Occult cancer
Cancer that is not detectable through standard physical exams; symptom-free disease.

Currently, the AUA does not recommend routine screening in men between ages 40 to 54 years at average risk. For men younger than age 55 years at higher risk, decisions regarding prostate cancer screening should be individualized.

---

care provider has not been obtaining PSA levels, then ask for a PSA test. Most insurance companies pay for prostate cancer screening. If yours doesn't, contact your local hospital or urologist's office to get the locations of free testing during Prostate Cancer Awareness Week (see Question 93).

28. When should I start worrying about prostate cancer?

Recent changes in the AUA guidelines (see Question 25) suggest that, in general, men concerned about prostate cancer risk and interested in prostate cancer screening, after discussing the benefits and risks, should start with screening when they're in their mid 50s. Men with a family history of prostate cancer and African American males should consider screening at a younger age. The American College of Surgeons (ACS) recommends discussing prostate cancer screening at 45 years of age for men at high risk, African Americans, and men with first-degree relatives (father, brother, or son) with prostate cancer diagnosed at < 65 years of age. The discussion should take place at 40 years of age for men at even higher risk (those with more than one first-degree relative who had prostate cancer at a younger age).

29. When should one stop having prostate cancer screening?

Prostate cancer screening is of maximal benefit for men who are going to live long enough to experience the benefits of treatment—which typically means men likely to live for at least ten years beyond the age at which they get a diagnosis of prostate cancer. Thus, if you have medical conditions that make survival of ten additional years less likely, you probably would not benefit from the early detection and treatment of prostate cancer and could stop prostate cancer screening. In addition, if you feel that you would not want any treatment for prostate cancer regardless of your age and overall health, then you should stop prostate cancer screening.

30. What is a digital rectal examination (DRE), and who should perform the DRE?

Because the prostate gland lies in front of the rectum, the back wall of the prostate gland can be felt by putting a gloved, lubricated finger into the rectum and feeling the prostate by pressing on the anterior wall of the rectum (**Figure 4**, page 35). The rectal examination allows one to feel only the back of the prostate. Ideally,

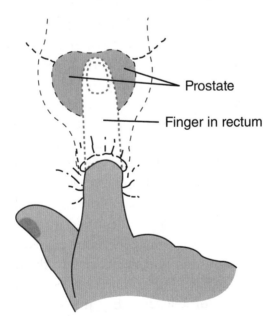

Prostate

Finger in rectum

Figure 4 Digital rectal examination of the prostate.

Data from *The Prostate Book: Sound Advice on Symptoms and Treatment*, Updated Edition by Stephen N. Rous, illustrated by Betty Goodwin. Copyright © 1992, 1988 by Stephen Rous.

the same doctor should perform the rectal examination each year so that the doctor is able to detect subtle changes in your prostate. The exam can be performed by a urologist or by an experienced primary care provider. If the primary care provider is concerned about your examination, you will be referred to a urologist.

31. I've had my rectum removed. How can my prostate be checked?

Traditionally, a prostate cancer screening involves a DRE and a serum PSA. The back surface of the prostate lies in front of the anterior surface (toward your abdomen) of the rectum; thus, pressing on the front surface of the rectum allows part of the prostate to be examined. There is no other way to physically examine the prostate. In men who have had their rectum removed for colorectal problems, such as cancer and certain inflammatory conditions, a rectal examination cannot be performed. In this situation, the physician must rely on the PSA level. If the PSA were to rise significantly, then a prostate biopsy should be performed. A transrectal ultrasound biopsy likewise cannot be performed in individuals without a rectum. In this situation, the biopsy is performed **transperineally**, which means through the **perineum** (the area under your scrotum). The ultrasound probe is placed in the area under the scrotum and in front of the expected location of the anus. The prostate is identified with the ultrasound probe, and then the needles are passed through the skin under ultrasound guidance into the different areas of the prostate. Performing biopsies this way can be more uncomfortable, and they are often performed with some form of anesthesia (general, spinal, or intravenous sedation).

Transperineal

Through the perineum.

Perineum

The area of the body that is behind the scrotum and in front of the anus.

32. What is a prostate nodule?

A prostate nodule is a firm, hard area in the prostate that feels like the knuckle of your finger. A prostate nodule may be cancerous and should be biopsied. Not all prostate nodules are cancers. Other causes of a nodule or a firm area in the prostate include prostatitis (prostate infection or inflammation), prostate calculi, an old **infarct** (an area of dead tissue resulting from a sudden loss of its blood supply) in the prostate, or abnormalities of the rectum, such as a hemorrhoid.

Infarct

An area of dead tissue resulting from a sudden loss of its blood supply.

33. If the PSA is increased, is the DRE always abnormal? And if the DRE is abnormal, is the PSA always abnormal?

When the PSA is increased, the rectal examination is not always abnormal. Remember that there are other causes of an increased PSA besides cancer. In addition, the rectal examination allows the doctor to examine only the back wall of the prostate, so some prostate cancers are not palpable by rectal examination. On the other hand, the PSA is not always increased when the rectal examination is abnormal. The PSA varies with the amount of prostate cancer present and with the grade of the cancer. In addition, a prostate nodule found during an examination is not always a cancer; it may be something in the wall of the rectum or may be related to prior inflammation or stones in the prostate. Further evaluation to rule out prostate cancer is indicated if either assessment (PSA or DRE) or both are abnormal.

34. If my PSA increases, do I need a biopsy done right away?

Because the PSA test is very sensitive and may be affected by inflammation or irritation of the prostate, the PSA value may fluctuate in some men who do not have cancer. If the rectal examination is normal, you can talk with your physician about repeating the PSA in six weeks to see whether it is returning to your baseline, or if this is your first PSA, to see whether it returns to a normal range. If it remains elevated or continues to increase, then a biopsy should be performed. Cancer cells do not sleep, they continue to grow, so there is no benefit to delaying the biopsy or subsequent treatment if the biopsy is positive. If the repeat PSA is decreasing, the PSA test could be repeated in 4 to 6 weeks, and monitoring could continue until the PSA normalizes or returns to your baseline.

35. What does a TRUS-guided prostate biopsy involve?

The transrectal ultrasound may be performed in your urologist's office or in the radiology department, depending on your institution. In preparation for the study, you may be asked to take an enema to clean stool out of the rectum and to take some antibiotics around the time of the study.

Some providers will have you come into the office approximately 2 weeks prior to your prostate biopsy to have a rectal swab culture. A small cotton swab-like instrument is placed into the rectum and the inside of the rectum is gently swiped. This is then sent for culture to determine if you have an antibiotic-resistant bacteria in the rectum. By doing this the provider can tailor the antibiotics prescribed and hopefully decrease the risk of a post-biopsy infection. Not all providers do this.

You will be asked to stop taking any aspirin or nonsteroidal anti-inflammatory medications, such as ibuprofen (Motrin or Advil) for about one week prior to the biopsy to minimize bleeding. The doctor will ask you to lie on your side with your legs bent and brought up to your abdomen. The ultrasound probe, which is a little larger than your thumb, is then gently placed into the rectum. This can cause some transient discomfort that usually stops when the probe is in place and completely goes away when the probe is removed. Men who have had prior rectal surgery, who have active hemorrhoids, or who are very anxious and cannot relax the external sphincter muscle may have more discomfort. Once the probe is in a good position, the prostate will be evaluated to make sure that there are no suspicious areas on the ultrasound.

An ultrasound looks at tissues by sound waves. The probe emits the sound waves, and the waves hit the prostate and are bounced off the prostate and surrounding tissue. The waves then return to the ultrasound probe, and a picture is developed on the screen. The sound waves do not cause any discomfort. Prostate cancer tends to cause less reflection of the sound waves, a trait referred to as **hypoechoic**, so the area often looks different in an ultrasound image than the normal prostate tissue. After the prostate has been evaluated, biopsies are obtained. The transrectal ultrasound allows the urologist to visualize the location for the biopsies. A minimum of six to eight biopsies are obtained and more frequently 12, distributed between the top, the bottom, and the middle aspect of the prostate on each side. If you have a large prostate gland, have suspicious areas

Hypoechoic

In ultrasonography, giving off few echoes; said of tissues or structures that reflect relatively few ultrasound waves directed at them.

on an ultrasound, or have had prior negative prostate biopsies, more biopsies may be obtained. Some providers will perform a nerve block, whereby lidocaine or a similar local anesthetic is injected on each side of the prostate prior to performing the biopsies.

MRI (magnetic resonance imaging) is used to help identify suspicious areas in the prostate and to guide prostate biopsy. A new technique, MRI/TRUS fusion biopsy, uses specialized software that fuses MRI images of the prostate with real-time ultrasound images of the prostate to provide the superior imaging of MRI with the ease of using the traditional ultrasound-guided prostate biopsy that can be done in the office.

Pathologist

A doctor trained in the evaluation of tissues under the microscope to determine the presence/absence of disease.

The Gleason grading system helps describe the appearance of the cancerous cells and may affect your prognosis.

Prognosis

The long-term outlook or prospect for survival and recovery from a disease.

36. Who decides that prostate cancer is present?

After your prostate biopsies have been obtained, they are sent to the **pathologist**, a doctor who specializes in the diagnosis of disease by studying cells and tissues under the microscope. The pathologist looks at the cells in the prostate biopsy specimens under the microscope to see if they appear normal or not. The pathologist may identify normal-appearing prostate cells, prostatitis (inflammation or infection of the prostate), benign prostatic enlargement, or cancerous cells. If cancerous cells are present, then the pathologist will look closely at the cells and assign a Gleason grade and score. The Gleason grading system helps describe the appearance of the cancerous cells and may affect your **prognosis** (the prediction made as to the outcome of your disease). In addition to the Gleason grade and score, the pathologist will also classify the prostate cancer according to the Gleason grade group.

37. Can the pathologist make a mistake in the diagnosis?

The use of a common grading system helps maintain uniformity in the grading of prostate cancer. The interobserver agreement (agreement between two different pathologists) and the intraobserver agreement (the same pathologist arriving at the same conclusion after reviewing the same slide twice) for the Gleason grading system are more than 80% and 90%, respectively. This means that two different pathologists reviewing the same slide agree on the Gleason grade for that slide 80% of the time, and that the same pathologist reviewing the same slide twice assigns the same grade to it both times 90% of the time.

The most frequent cause of differences in grading is the grading of tumors that vary between two grades. A Gleason sum of 2 to 4 is uncommon and should be found only in a small number of needle biopsy specimens. It is the Gleason sum of 2 to 4 that tends to be upgraded to a higher sum a small percentage of the time when reviewed by another pathologist. There is a tendency for the needle biopsy Gleason grade to be lower than the pathologic grade at the time of radical prostatectomy. This difference in Gleason grade probably reflects the presence of a higher-grade cancer in another area of the prostate that had not been biopsied at the time of the prostate biopsy. It is very rare for the pathologist to say that there is no cancer in the specimen and for another pathologist to state that there is. (Similarly, it is rare for one pathologist to say that cancer is present and another pathologist to state that it is not present.)

38. What is the Gleason grade/score?

Gleason grade/ score

A newer technique to stratify prostate cancer risk, 5 categories.

Gleason scale

A commonly used method to classify how cells appear in cancerous tissues; the less the cancerous cells look like normal cells, the more malignant the cancer; two numbers, each from 1 to 5, are assigned to the two most predominant types of cells present. These two numbers are added together to produce the Gleason score. Higher numbers indicate more aggressive cancers.

The grade of a cancer is a term used to describe how the cancer cells look; that is, whether the cells look aggressive and not very similar to normal cells (high grade) or whether they look very similar to normal cells (low grade). The grade of the cancer is an important factor in predicting long-term results of treatment, response to treatment, and survival. With prostate cancer, the most commonly used grading system is the **Gleason scale**. In this grading system, cells are examined by a pathologist under the microscope and assigned a number based on how the cancer cells look and how they are arranged together (**Figure 5**, page 43). Because prostate cancer may be composed of cancer cells of different grades, the pathologist assigns numbers to the two predominant grades present. The numbers range from 1 (low grade) to 5 (high grade). Typically, the Gleason score is the total of these two numbers; for example, a man with a Gleason grade of 2 and 3 in his prostate cancer would have a Gleason score of 5. An exception to this occurs where the highest (most aggressive) pattern present in a biopsy is neither the most predominant nor the second most predominant pattern. In this situation, the Gleason score is obtained by combining the most predominant pattern grade with the highest grade. Occasionally, if a small component of a tumor on prostatectomy is of a pattern that is higher than the two most predominant patterns, then the minor component is noted as a tertiary grade to the pathology report.

Lower-risk prostate cancer is a Gleason score less than or equal to 6. Intermediate risk is a Gleason score of 7. High risk is a Gleason score of 8–10. The higher the Gleason score, the more aggressive the cancer. Gleason scores 8 through 10 are highly aggressive tumors that are often difficult to cure. Sometimes these cancers are so abnormal that they do not even produce PSA. The grade of the cancer identified by the biopsies may differ from the grade that is present in the entire prostate, because it is possible that the biopsy may not identify areas of higher-grade cancers.

More recently a 5 grade scoring system has been adopted for prostate cancer. Gleason grade group 1 applies to those biopsies where the Gleason score is 6 or less. Gleason grade group 2 applies to biopsy specimens that have both

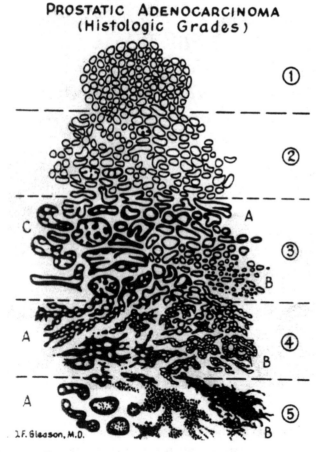

Figure 5 Gleason grading system of prostate adenocarcinoma.

Reprinted with permission from Walsh PC, Stamey TA, Retik AB, and Vaughan, ED, Jr, eds. *Campbell's Urology*, 7th ed., Copyright Elsevier 1997.

Gleason 3 and 4 present (Gleason score of 7), however, the most prominent grade is 3. Gleason grade group 3 applies to biopsy specimens that have both Gleason 3 and 4 (Gleason score of 7), however, the grade 4 prostate cancer is more prominent in the biopsy specimen. Gleason grade group 4 applies to a Gleason score of 8. Gleason grade group 5 applies to a Gleason score of 9–10.

39. I recently had a prostate biopsy that showed no prostate cancer cells, but my doctor tells me I need a repeat biopsy because I have PIN. What is PIN, and why do I need a repeat biopsy? What are atypical glands suspicious for prostate cancer? Do I need a repeat biopsy with this finding?

Prostatic intraepithelial neoplasia (PIN)

An abnormal area in a prostate biopsy specimen that is not cancerous, but may become cancerous or be associated with cancer elsewhere in the prostate.

PIN is the abbreviation for **prostatic intraepithelial neoplasia**. PIN is identified by the pathologist examining the prostate biopsies. PIN has been thought to be a precancerous lesion. More recently, PIN has been divided into two types, low-grade PIN and high-grade PIN, based on how the cells look. Low-grade PIN does not appear to have any increased risk of prostate cancer. High-grade PIN, however, is often found in association with prostate cancer. In 35–45% of men who undergo a repeat biopsy for high-grade PIN, prostate cancer cells are present in the repeat biopsy. No current method can discriminate which high-grade PIN lesions will progress to clinically significant prostate cancer versus a less aggressive prostate cancer. The Canadian Urologic Association argues that in the current era of extended (greater number) biopsy schemes, high-grade PIN (HGPIN) is no longer considered a strict indication for repeat biopsy and patients should be followed clinically with PSA and DRE. The current NCCN guidelines for high-grade PIN differentiate between multifocal (present in 2 or more areas in the biopsy specimen) and focal (one area). If there is multifocal PIN, it is recommended that one consider serum or urine biomarkers (see Table 1, page 10) and/or multiparametric MRI and consider re-biopsy with increased sampling. *Atypical gland; suspicious for cancer* is noted on the pathology report when the pathologist sees an atypical area that has most of the features of cancer, but a definitive diagnosis of cancer cannot be made due to the small size of the area and the small number of abnormal cells present. Repeat biopsy in patients with this diagnosis have up to a 60% chance of having prostate cancer present in a repeat biopsy. Thus, the finding of atypical gland; suspicious for cancer requires further evaluation. The NCCN guidelines recommend consideration of (1) urine or serum biomarkers and/or multiparametric MRI and (2) consider repeat biopsy with increased sampling in the area of the prostate where the atypical cells were noted on the initial biopsy (NCCN guidelines version 1.2018. Prostate Cancer Early Detection. www.NCCN.org). If no cancer is found on the repeat biopsy, then close follow-up with PSA, DRE, and periodic biopsy may be needed.

40. I just had a TURP, and my doctor called and told me that there is cancer in the specimen. Will the TURP cause my cancer to spread? Will it prevent me from having certain treatments for prostate cancer?

Before the identification of PSA, prostate cancer was detected by a palpable nodule on DRE, the presence of metastatic disease, or transurethral resection of the prostate, also called transurethral prostatectomy (TURP). TURP is one of the most common forms of surgical therapy for BPH. The procedure uses an instrument called a resectoscope (similar to a telescope—it has an eyepiece, a lens, and a light source), which is passed through the urethra. The prostatic tissue that is bulging into the urethra and blocking the outflow of urine is cut away (resected) using a special loop that is connected to an electrical current. The resection is continued until it appears that all of the obstructing prostate tissue is removed. The prostate tissue, called "chips," is then removed through the scope and sent to the pathologist for examination under a microscope.

Similar to the procedure with needle biopsies of the prostate, if the pathologist identifies cancer cells in the specimen, he or she grades the prostate cancer cells and determines a Gleason score. The pathologist also determines what percentage of the prostate chips have cancer present in them. Typically, if less than 5% of the chips contain cancer and the Gleason score is low (< 6), then the prostate cancer is considered to be clinically insignificant, and you can be followed with DREs and PSA tests. If more than 5% of the tissue contains prostate cancer and/or the Gleason score is high, the cancer is considered to be potentially aggressive and warrants further treatment. Similar to any newly diagnosed prostate cancer, it is important to determine the clinical stage of the cancer and to assess whether the cancer is likely to be confined to the prostate through the use of nomograms (**Table 5**, pages 48–52), and staging studies, such as a bone scan, if indicated.

The TURP does not cause the prostate cancer to spread, nor does it make it easier for the cancer cells to spread. However, the TURP can affect the risks of future treatments for prostate cancer. A TURP makes interstitial seed therapy more difficult to perform and is associated with a much higher risk of urinary incontinence, making it less desirable. Radical prostatectomy and external-beam radiation therapy can be performed after TURP without an increased risk.

Table 5 Nomograms Predicting Pathologic Stage of CaP Based on Clinical Stage (TNM), PSA, and Gleason Score

PSA Range (ng/mL)	Pathologic Stage	Biopsy Gleason Score			
		5–6	3 + 4 = 7	4 + 3 = 7	8–10
Clinical Stage T1c (nonpalpable, PSA elevated) n = 4419					
0–2.5	Organ confined (n = 226)	93 (91–95)	82 (76–87)	73 (64–80)	77 (65–85)
	Extraprostatic extension (n = 19)	6 (5–8)	14 (10–18)	20 (14–28)	16 (11–24)
	Seminal vesicle (+) (n = 1)	0 (0–1)	2 (0–5)	2 (0–5)	3 (0–8)
	Lymph node (+) (n = 3)	0 (0–1)	2 (0–6)	4 (1–12)	3 (1–12)
2.6–4.0	Organ confined (n = 619)	88 (86–90)	72 (67–76)	61 (54–68)	66 (57–74)
	Extraprostatic extension (n = 92)	11 (10–13)	23 (19–27)	33 (27–39)	26 (19–34)
	Seminal vesicle (+) (n = 8)	1 (0–1)	4 (2–7)	5 (2–8)	7 (3–13)
	Lymph node (+) (n = 1)	0 (0–0)	1 (0–1)	1 (0–3)	1 (0–3)
4.1–6.0	Organ confined (n = 1266)	83 (81–85)	63 (59–67)	51 (45–56)	55 (46–64)
	Extraprostatic extension (n = 297)	16 (14–17)	30 (26–33)	40 (34–45)	32 (25–40)
	Seminal vesicle (+) (n = 37)	1 (1–1)	6 (4–8)	7 (4–10)	10 (6–15)
	Lymph node (+) (n = 12)	0 (0–0)	2 (1–3)	3 (1–6)	3 (1–6)

PSA Range (ng/mL)	Pathologic Stage	Biopsy Gleason Score			
		5–6	3 + 4 = 7	4 + 3 = 7	8–10
6.1–10.0	Organ confined (n = 989)	81 (79–83)	59 (54–64)	47 (41–53)	51 (41–59)
	Extraprostatic extension (n = 281)	18 (16–19)	32 (27–36)	42 (36–47)	34 (26–42)
	Seminal vesicle (+) (n = 36)	1 (1–2)	8 (6–11)	8 (5–12)	12 (8–19)
	Lymph node (+) (n = 5)	0 (0–0)	1 (1–3)	3 (1–5)	3 (1–5)
> 10.0	Organ confined (n = 324)	70 (66–74)	42 (37–48)	30 (25–36)	34 (26–42)
	Extraprostatic extension (n = 165)	27 (23–30)	40 (35–45)	48 (40–55)	39 (31–48)
	Seminal vesicle (+) (n = 25)	2 (2–3)	12 (8–16)	11 (7–17)	17 (10–25)
	Lymph node (+) (n = 13)	1 (0–1)	6 (3–9)	10 (5–17)	9 (4–17)
Clinical Stage T2a (palpable < ½ of one lobe) (n = 998)					
0–2.5	Organ confined (n = 156)	88 (84–90)	70 (63–77)	58 (48–67)	63 (51–74)
	Extraprostatic extension (n = 18)	12 (9–15)	24 (18–30)	32 (24–41)	26 (18–36)
	Seminal vesicle (+) (n = 2)	0 (0–1)	2 (0–6)	3 (0–7)	4 (0–10)
	Lymph node (+) (n = 1)	0 (0–1)	3 (1–9)	7 (1–17)	6 (1–16)

(continues)

Table 5 Nomograms Predicting Pathologic Stage of CaP Based on Clinical Stage (TNM), PSA, and Gleason Score (continued)

PSA Range (ng/mL)	Pathologic Stage	Biopsy Gleason Score				
		5–6	3 + 4 = 7	4 + 3 = 7	8–10	
2.6–4.0	Organ confined (n = 124)	79 (75–82)	57 (51–63)	45 (38–52)	50 (40–59)	
	Extraprostatic extension (n = 49)	20 (17–24)	37 (31–42)	48 (40–55)	40 (30–50)	
	Seminal vesicle (+) (n = 5)	1 (0–1)	5 (3–9)	5 (3–10)	8 (4–15)	
	Lymph node (+) (n = 0)	0 (0–0)	1 (0–2)	2 (0–5)	2 (0–4)	
4.1–6.0	Organ confined (n = 171)	71 (67–75)	47 (41–52)	34 (28–41)	39 (31–48)	
	Extraprostatic extension (n = 101)	27 (23–31)	44 (39–49)	54 (47–60)	46 (37–54)	
	Seminal vesicle (+) (n = 10)	1 (1–2)	7 (4–10)	7 (4–11)	11 (6–17)	
	Lymph node (+) (n = 3)	0 (0–1)	2 (1–4)	5 (2–8)	4 (2–9)	
6.1–10.0	Organ confined (n = 142)	68 (64–72)	43 (38–48)	31 (26–37)	36 (27–44)	
	Extraprostatic extension (n = 99)	29 (26–33)	46 (41–51)	56 (49–62)	47 (37–56)	
	Seminal vesicle (+) (n = 12)	2 (1–3)	9 (6–13)	9 (5–14)	13 (8–20)	
	Lymph node (+) (n = 6)	0 (1–0)	2 (1–4)	4 (2–8)	4 (1–8)	

PSA Range (ng/mL)	Pathologic Stage	Biopsy Gleason Score			
		5–6	3 + 4 = 7	4 + 3 = 7	8–10
> 10.0	Organ confined (n = 36)	54 (49–60)	28 (23–33)	18 (14–23)	21 (15–28)
	Extraprostatic extension (n = 47)	41 (35–46)	52 (46–59)	57 (48–66)	49 (39–59)
	Seminal vesicle (+) (n = 9)	3 (2–5)	12 (7–18)	11 (6–17)	17 (9–25)
	Lymph node (+) (n = 7)	1 (0–3)	7 (3–14)	13 (6–24)	12 (5–22)
Clinical Stage T2b (palpable ≥ ½ of lobe) or T2c (palpable both lobes) (n = 313)					
0–2.5	Organ confined (n = 16)	84 (78–89)	59 (47–70)	44 (31–58)	49 (32–65)
	Extraprostatic extension (n = 10)	14 (9–19)	24 (16–33)	29 (19–42)	24 (14–36)
	Seminal vesicle (+) (n = 0)	1 (0–3)	6 (0–14)	6 (0–14)	8 (0–21)
	Lymph node (+) (n = 0)	1 (0–3)	10 (2–25)	19 (4–40)	17 (3–42)
2.6–4.0	Organ confined (n = 28)	74 (68–80)	47 (39–56)	36 (27–45)	39 (28–50)
	Extraprostatic extension (n = 15)	23 (18–29)	37 (28–45)	46 (36–55)	37 (27–48)
	Seminal vesicle (+) (n = 3)	2 (1–5)	13 (7–21)	13 (7–22)	19 (9–32)
	Lymph node (+) (n = 2)	0 (0–1)	3 (0–7)	5 (0–14)	4 (0–13)

(continues)

Table 5 Nomograms Predicting Pathologic Stage of CaP Based on Clinical Stage (TNM), PSA, and Gleason Score (continued)

PSA Range (ng/mL)	Pathologic Stage	Biopsy Gleason Score			
		5–6	3 + 4 = 7	4 + 3 = 7	8–10
4.1–6.0	Organ confined (n = 46)	66 (59–72)	36 (29–43)	25 (19–32)	27 (19–37)
	Extraprostatic extension (n = 40)	30 (24–36)	41 (33–47)	47 (38–55)	38 (28–48)
	Seminal vesicle (+) (n = 7)	4 (2–6)	16 (10–23)	15 (9–23)	22 (13–33)
	Lymph node (+) (n = 4)	1 (0–2)	7 (3–12)	13 (6–21)	11 (4–23)
6.1–10.0	Organ confined (n = 53)	62 (55–68)	32 (26–38)	22 (17–29)	24 (17–33)
	Extraprostatic extension (n = 28)	32 (26–38)	41 (33–49)	47 (38–56)	38 (29–48)
	Seminal vesicle (+) (n = 15)	5 (3–8)	20 (13–28)	19 (11–28)	27 (16–39)
	Lymph node (+) (n = 5)	1 (0–2)	6 (3–11)	11 (5–19)	10 (3–20)
> 10.0	Organ confined (n = 8)	46 (39–53)	18 (13–24)	11 (7–15)	12 (7–18)
	Extraprostatic extension (n = 15)	41 (34–50)	40 (31–51)	40 (30–52)	33 (22–46)
	Seminal vesicle (+) (n = 10)	7 (4–12)	23 (15–33)	19 (10–29)	28 (16–42)
	Lymph node (+) (n = 8)	5 (2–8)	18 (9–30)	29 (15–44)	26 (12–44)

Makarov DV, et al. *Urology* 2007; 69(6): 1095–1101.

PART FOUR

Prostate Cancer Staging

How does one know if the prostate cancer
is confined to the prostate?

How and why does one stage prostate cancer?

What is a bone scan?

More . . .

41. How does one know if the prostate cancer is confined to the prostate?

By staging your cancer, your doctor is trying to assess, based on your prostate biopsy results, your physical examination, your PSA, and other tests and X-rays (if obtained), whether your prostate cancer is confined to the prostate, and if it is not, to what extent it has spread. Studies of large numbers of men who have undergone radical prostatectomy and pelvic lymph node dissections have established some guidelines regarding the likelihood of prostate capsular involvement and lymph node metastases (Table 5, pages 48–52). It was initially thought that magnetic resonance imaging (MRI) would be very helpful in determining whether capsular penetration and extracapsular disease were present; however, it has only proved to be useful in centers that perform large numbers of MRIs. Similarly, the use of computed tomographic (CT) scanning in assessing whether or not the cancer has spread to the pelvic lymph nodes has been disappointing (see Question 42). CT is rarely positive when the PSA is less than 20 ng/mL. The sensitivity of a CT scan for detecting positive lymph nodes is only 30–35% at a PSA greater than 25 ng/mL. CT is used in the initial staging of select patients with T3 or T4 disease and patients with T1 or T2 disease with nomogram indicated probability of lymph node involvement that is greater than 10%. An MRI can be used in the staging and characterization of prostate cancer and may be used to better risk stratify men considering active surveillance. Another study, a bone scan (Question 43) and plain X-ray, if needed, is used to determine if the prostate cancer has spread to the bones.

42. How and why does one stage prostate cancer?

Knowing the stage (the size and the extent of spread) of the prostate cancer helps the doctor counsel you on treatment options. Your doctor may tell you a "clinical" stage, based on your rectal examination, prostate biopsies (**Figure 6**, page 55), and radiographic/nuclear medicine studies (CT scan, bone scan, MRI). Pathological staging is performed when a pathologist examines the prostate, seminal vesicles, and pelvic lymph nodes (if removed) at the time of radical prostatectomy. The most common staging system used is called the **TNM System**. In this

DIAGNOSIS

TNM System

The most common staging system for prostate cancer. It reflects the size of the tumor, nodal disease, and metastatic disease.

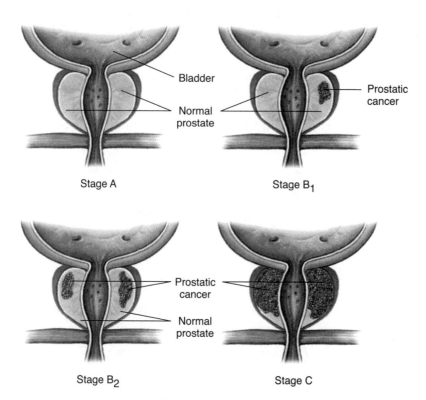

Figure 6 The prostate gland showing the different stages of cancer.

Data from *The Prostate Book: Sound Advice on Symptoms and Treatment*, Updated Edition by Stephen N. Rous, illustrated by Betty Goodwin. Copyright © 1992, 1988 by Stephen Rous.

system, *T* refers to the size of the tumor in the prostate, *N* refers to the extent of cancerous involvement of the lymph nodes, and *M* refers to the presence or absence of **metastases** (deposits of prostate cancer outside of the prostate and lymph nodes) (*AJCC Cancer Staging Manual*, 8th ed., 2017).

Metastases

Deposits of prostate cancer outside of the prostate and lymph nodes.

T   Refers to the size of the tumor in the prostate

T1 The prostate cancer is located within the prostate and cannot be palpated on rectal examination

    T1a: tumor is found incidentally in < 5% of the prostate tissue, such as during a TURP

    T1b: tumor is found incidentally in > 5% of the prostate tissue, such as during a TURP

    T1c: prostate cancer is identified by needle biopsy for an increased PSA

T2 The prostate cancer is still located in the prostate and the tumor is large enough to be felt on rectal examination

    T2a: tumor involves half of a lobe or less

    T2b: tumor involves one lobe

    T2c: tumor involves both lobes

T3 The tumor extends through the prostate capsule

    T3a: tumor has spread outside of the prostate capsule, unilateral or bilateral; microscopic bladder neck invasion

    T3b: tumor invades seminal vesicle

T4 The tumor is fixed or invades adjacent structures other than seminal vesicles, such as bladder neck, external sphincter, rectum, levator muscles, and/or pelvic wall

N   Describes the extent of lymph node involvement

    N0: no evidence of any metastases in the pelvic lymph nodes

    N1: prostate cancer cells found in a single, small (< 2 cm) lymph node

    N1: metastases in nearby lymph node(s)

    N1: metastases in regional lymph node(s)

M   Refers to the presence or absence of metastases

    M0: no evidence of distant metastases (tumor outside of the pelvis)

    M1: distant metastases (tumor spread outside of the pelvis to other areas of the body, such as bones, liver)

Histopatholic Grade G

    Gx: grade cannot be assessed

    G1: Gleason score 2–4

    G2: Gleason score 5–6

    G3: Gleason score 7–10

Prostate Cancer Stage Groupings

    Stage I T1a, N0, M0, G1

    Stage II T1a, N0, M0, G2–4
              T1b, N0, M0, any G
              T1, N0, M0, any G
              T2, N0 M0, any G

    Stage III T3, N0, M0, any G

    Stage IV T4, N0, M0, any G
              any T, N1, M0, any G
              any T, any N, M1, any G

Data from: *www.auanet.org/guidelines*

43. What is a bone scan? Are there other tests to determine if the prostate cancer has spread to the bones?

Bone scan

A specialized nuclear medicine study that allows one to detect changes in the bone that may be related to metastatic prostate cancer.

A **bone scan** is a study performed in the nuclear medicine department that involves injecting a small amount of a radioactive chemical through a vein into your bloodstream. The chemical circulates through your body and is picked up by areas of fast bone growth that may be associated with cancer. Technetium-99m radionuclide bone scan is the most cost-effective and available whole-body screening test for the evaluation of bone metastases. A plain X-ray is the best method to evaluate areas that are suspicious on bone scan. The bone scan is the most sensitive technique currently available for identifying prostate cancer that has spread to the bones (**Figure 7**, page 59). Other problems of the bones, such as a history of a broken bone, arthritis, and a condition called Paget's disease, may cause an increase in uptake of the radioactive chemical. Often, your history, the location of the bone, and possible additional studies, such as a plain X-ray study or an MRI, will help determine whether the area of increased uptake indicates the presence of cancer.

Osteoblastic lesion

Pertaining to plain X-ray of a bone, increased density of bone seen on X-ray when there is extensive new bone formation due to cancerous destruction of the bone.

The bone scan is quite sensitive, but it does not identify small numbers of cancer cells in the bones. In a small number of men (8%), the bone scan may be normal when bone metastases are present. Prostate cancer is not the only cancer that spreads to the bone, but prostate cancer tends to cause the bone to look different than that of involvement with other cancers, such as breast, colon, and bladder. Prostate cancer metastases are typically osteoblastic, whereas those of other cancers tend to be osteolytic. **Osteoblastic lesions** look as if there is an increase in the amount of bone present on a plain X-ray, whereas **osteolytic lesions** look like there is a loss of

Osteolytic lesion

Pertaining to plain X-ray of a bone, refers to decreased density of bone seen on X-ray when there is destruction and loss of bone by cancer.

bone. The bone scan may also show an obstruction of the urinary tract, leading to hydronephrosis (a back-up of urine in the kidney that causes swelling of the kidney).

The bone scan is often obtained as part of the staging work-up in men with prostate cancer and is helpful in men with a rising PSA (either after primary treatment, such as radical prostatectomy, or during watchful waiting) with or without bone pain to identify new areas of uptake that may indicate new bone involvement. The AUA guidelines recommend considering an initial bone scan for patients with one or more of the following: PSA greater than or equal to 20 ng/mL, clinical stage T3a or higher, Gleason score greater than or equal to 8, or bone pain. Although the chemical used for the study is radioactive, the amount used is small, and it will not put you or your family at risk.

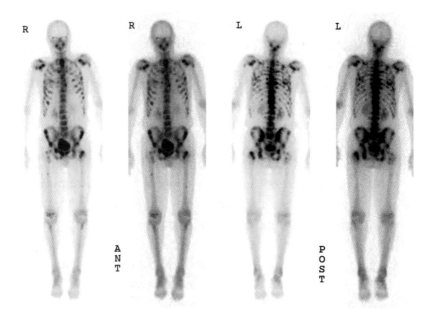

Figure 7 Bone scan used to detect prostate cancer metastases.
© Steven Needell/Science Source

CT and MRI are useful in evaluating suspicious areas on a bone scan that appear equivocal on a plain X-ray. MRI can help detect metastatic areas in the bone before they are detectable on a bone scan. However, an MRI is 2–3 times more costly than a bone scan. Positron emission tomography (PET) scans using an injection of various radioactively labeled chemicals appear to be more sensitive and specific for bone metastases than bone scans, but are around 8 times more costly than a bone scan.

44. What is a pelvic lymph node dissection and what are the risks?

The first location to which prostate cancer tends to spread if it goes outside of the prostate is the pelvic lymph nodes. It is important to know whether the cancer has spread to the lymph nodes because the success rates of treatments such as interstitial seed therapy and radical prostatectomy are lower if the cancer has spread into the pelvic lymph nodes. Thus, the urologist or radiation oncologist should have a good idea whether there is prostate cancer involvement of the pelvic lymph nodes before recommending a therapy. Unfortunately, radiologic studies such as CT scans have not been helpful in identifying individuals with smaller amounts of cancer in the pelvic lymph nodes. The most accurate way to assess the lymph node status is to remove the lymph nodes and have them examined by the pathologist. The lymph nodes to which prostate cancer typically spreads are located in the lateral aspect of each side of the pelvis (see Question 22). Removing the lymph nodes requires surgery, either an open procedure or a laparoscopic procedure, which has risks. Not everyone needs a pelvic lymph node dissection. When the risk of having positive lymph nodes is low, such as occurs in men with a low Gleason score, < 6, or a PSA > 10, a lymph node dissection is unnecessary, and one can proceed directly with definitive therapy, such as interstitial seed therapy, external beam radiation therapy (EBRT), and radical prostatectomy (see **Part 5**) for descriptions of these therapies). In high-risk patients, those with higher Gleason scores (8–10), or those with a PSA > 10, a lymph node dissection may be performed at the same time as a planned radical prostatectomy or before planned EBRT or interstitial seed therapy. If a radical prostatectomy (open, laparoscopic, robotic) is planned, the lymph nodes can be removed using the same approach as for the prostatectomy and can be examined by the pathologist (frozen section) just before the surgeon performs the prostatectomy. Frozen section specimens are interpreted by the pathologist shortly after they are removed from the patient, and the findings are reported to the surgeon in the operating room.

The surgeon then decides whether to proceed with removal of the prostate based on whether cancer has been identified in the lymph nodes. Some surgeons remove the prostate in the presence of small amounts of cancer in the lymph nodes, whereas others do not. The slides are then made into permanent sections and reviewed again by the pathologist. In most cases, the interpretation of the frozen section is the same as that of the permanent section; rarely do the two differ. In a perineal prostatectomy, the perineal incision does not allow access to the pelvic lymph nodes, and a separate midline incision or a laparoscopic approach is needed for the lymph node dissection. With EBRT or interstitial seed therapy, the pelvic lymph node dissection may be performed laparoscopically or via an open incision that is located below the umbilicus on a separate day before EBRT/interstitial seeds.

A lymph node dissection should be performed in high-risk patients because it may affect treatment. The likelihood of having positive nodes varies with the stage of the prostate cancer, the PSA value, and the Gleason score. Approximately 5–12% of men who are believed to have clinically localized prostate cancer (low stage) have cancer that has spread to the pelvic lymph nodes. Before the pelvic lymph node dissection, you should discuss with your doctor how your planned prostate cancer treatment would be affected if you had cancer involving the pelvic lymph nodes.

The main risks of a pelvic lymph node dissection are bleeding, nerve injury, and **lymphocele**.

Lymphocele

A collection of lymph fluid in an area of the body.

- *Bleeding*: The nodes that are removed at the time of the pelvic lymph node dissection surround some large pelvic arteries and veins, called the iliac vessels. Injury to these vessels or their branches may cause bleeding. It is rare to have a significant blood loss such that a blood transfusion would be required.

- *Nerve injury*: The obturator nerve supplies muscles in the leg and is surrounded by some of the pelvic lymph nodes. If the nerve is cut or damaged at the time of surgery and the damage is recognized, it may be sewn back together. If the injury is not recognized, it may lead to a permanent inability to cross your leg on the side of the injury.

- *Lymphocele*: A lymphocele is a collection of lymph fluid that accumulates in the pelvis. Lymphoceles result from an injury to the lymph vessels. When the lymph nodes are being removed, the lymphatic vessels are clipped, tied, or cauterized to minimize leakage of lymph fluid from the vessel. A lymphocele may go undetected and may not cause any harm. If the lymphocele gets large enough, it may put pressure on other tissues and cause abdominal pressure or pain. If the lymphocele becomes infected, you may develop a fever or chills and abdominal pain. Lymphoceles are identified in one to two of every 100 men undergoing radical prostatectomy. The actual incidence may be higher with smaller lymphoceles that do not cause any symptoms and thus are not identified. Treatment of a lymphocele varies with its size and symptoms. If the lymphocele is small and does not cause any symptoms, it can be monitored to see whether it will go away on its own. If the lymphocele is large and causes symptoms or if it is infected, then it should be drained. Usually, a radiologist is able to pass a small drainage tube through the skin into the area where the lymphocele is located to drain the fluid. The drain is left in place until there is no further drainage and an ultrasound or CT scan shows that the lymphocele has resolved. In most patients, this is all that is needed. Rarely, the lymphocele recurs, requiring repeat drainage or surgery.

45. Are there other radiologic studies used in the evaluation of prostate cancer?

Positron emission tomography (PET)/CT is a nuclear medicine study that allows for the simultaneous performance of two different types of imaging studies. It involves a PET scanner and a CT scanner. Images from both of these studies are combined to provide a functional (metabolic or biological activity) and anatomic evaluation of the areas of the body. The use of C-11 choline tracers in PET/CT may help identify sites of metastases in men with biochemical recurrence of prostate cancer after primary treatment and lymph node metastases. Another agent that is being evaluated is 18F-fluoride.

The role of an MRI in prostate cancer continues to evolve. MRI has been shown to have a role in the detection of prostate cancer, assisting with targeting of the area in the prostate to biopsy (targeting) and staging of prostate cancer. An MRI can be coupled with an ultrasound to enhance the detection and localization of prostate cancer, but still allow the prostate biopsy to be performed in the office (see Question 35). With respect to the staging of prostate cancer, an MRI has been shown to be helpful in the identification of patients extension of the prostate cancer outside of the prostate capsule (extracapsular extension) as well as extension into the nerves surrounding the prostate (neurovascular bundles), seminal vesicles, and other structures such as the bladder or rectum. This additional information is helpful in determining if an individual truly has localized prostate cancer (cancer confined to the prostate), which may affect treatment decisions and outcomes. An MRI has also been demonstrated to help determine local recurrence of prostate cancer after radical prostatectomy and radiation therapy. In addition, the use of an MRI may be helpful to better risk stratify men with prostate cancer considering active surveillance.

A combination of a bone scan and a single photon emission computed tomography (SPECT) is a way to improve the sensitivity and specificity of a bone scan. During a SPECT scan, the camera rotates around the body, taking pictures as it rotates, as opposed to a regular bone scan, in which the camera passes straight over the body. The addition of SPECT allows one to see smaller areas in detail.

PART FIVE

Treatment of Prostate Cancer

Why do I need a team of doctors to treat me?
Who are they?

What options do I have for treatment
of my prostate cancer?

What are castrate-resistant prostate cancer (CRPC)
and metastatic castrate-resistant prostate cancer
(mCRPC), and how are they treated?

More . . .

46. Why do I need a team of doctors to treat me? Who are they?

Cancer is a complex disease, and understanding and treating it requires knowledge of genetics, molecular biology, pharmacology, radiation therapy, nutrition, surgery, and other essential information. No one doctor is able to provide all of the care and service you may need, so it's necessary that a team of specialists look at your case from the perspective of each clinician's area of expertise. This multidisciplinary approach will ensure that you have access to all of the treatment options available.

The following doctors are likely to play a role on your team:

Urologist

A doctor that specializes in the evaluation and treatment of diseases of the genito-urinary tract in men and women.

Urologist: A urologist specializes in the diagnosis and treatment of disorders of the genito-urinary system. Your urologist probably diagnosed your prostate cancer and helped you plan your course of treatment. This physician has likely been overseeing all of your procedures and program of therapy.

Radiation oncologist

A physician who treats cancer through the use of radiation therapy.

Radiation oncologist: This type of doctor treats cancer through radiation, or high-energy rays. You might have received radiation therapy from a radiation oncologist in the form of external beam radiation or brachytherapy. External beam radiation directs X-rays from a machine at the prostate gland. Brachytherapy consists of tiny radioactive seeds placed inside or near the tumor (see Question 47).

Medical oncologist

See **oncologist**.

Medical oncologist: If prostate cancer reappears despite surgery or no longer responds to hormonal therapy, a medical oncologist should join the treatment team because he or she may use chemotherapy, immunotherapy, and alternative therapies that affect hormone production/action. A medical oncologist is a doctor who specializes in treating patients diagnosed with cancer. He or she helps you plan chemotherapy or other therapies and takes charge of these treatments. The medical oncologist may also make recommendations regarding clinical trials (see Question 89).

47. What options do I have for treatment of my prostate cancer?

Cliff's comment:

After finally realizing that despite feeling great, I did indeed have prostate cancer, I had to figure out what the best treatment for me was. When faced with the option of leaving my prostate in place or removing it, I knew that, even though I was petrified of surgery, it would be the best thing for me in the long run. I knew that I could not live with my prostate gland and the continuous question of whether there were any viable cancer cells remaining in my prostate after interstitial seeds or radiation therapy.

Various treatment options are available for prostate cancer, each with its own risks and benefits (**Table 6**, pages 68–71). The options available may vary with the grade of tumor, the extent of tumor spread, your overall medical health and life expectancy, and your personal preferences. The treatments for prostate cancer can be divided into those that are intended to "cure" your cancer (definitive therapies) and those that are **palliative**, intended to slow down the growth of the prostate cancer and treat its symptoms. Definitive therapies for localized prostate cancer include: interstitial seed therapy (brachytherapy), external beam radiation (EBRT), and radical prostatectomy (either open, laparoscopic, or robot-assisted). Other therapies, such as cryotherapy, high-intensity focused ultrasound (HIFU), and combination therapy (external beam radiation plus

TREATMENT OF PROSTATE CANCER

Palliative

Treatment designed to relieve a particular problem without necessarily solving it; e.g., palliative therapy is given in order to relieve symptoms and improve quality of life, but it does not cure the patient.

The treatments for prostate cancer can be divided into those that are intended to "cure" your cancer (definitive therapies) and those that are palliative, intended to slow down the growth of the prostate cancer and treat its symptoms.

Table 6 Initial Treatment Options for Prostate Cancer

Mode of Treatment	Advantages	Disadvantages	Curative: Yes/No	Alternative If Fails
Hormonal therapy • Therapy that prevents the production of male hormones (androgens). • Primary treatment for older men with prostate cancer who don't want surgery or forms of XRT but also don't want to watch and wait.	1. *Orchiectomy:* A one-time procedure that avoids the need for shots; it drops testosterone quickly to almost zero and is permanent. 2. *GnRH agonists/antagonist:* Not permanent.	1. *Orchiectomy:* Permanent outpatient procedure involves minor surgery, risk of infection, bleeding, pain. 2. *GnRH agonist:* Can have flair of bone pain in those with bone metastases; need to pretreat these men with androgen receptor blocker; requires monthly to yearly visits or shots, which can be expensive. GnRH antagonist—avoids flair of bone pain, but is currently only available as an every 1 month injection.	No: hormone therapy slows the growth of those prostate cancer cells that are hormone sensitive. Used for treatment of metastatic disease.	Chemotherapy Immunotherapy and alternative therapies that affect testosterone production/action.
Cryotherapy/Surgery	Minimally invasive, no blood loss. Quicker recovery; one-time procedure; can be used in those who cannot undergo RRPX or as salvage procedure for local recurrence after XRT.	Impotence, urethral strictures, urinary retention, urinary frequency, dysuria, hematuria, penile or scrotal swelling, fistula, incomplete treatment of cancer. Works better on smaller prostates; more difficult to perform if prior TURP (transurethral resection of prostate); incontinence up to 30% when used as salvage procedure.	Role is not well defined; this therapy is being used primarily for XRT failures, but some have used it as first line.	Hormone treatment, radical prostatectomy, but there is increased risk of complications.

Mode of Treatment	Advantages	Disadvantages	Curative: Yes/No	Alternative If Fails
Radical retropubic prostatectomy with/without bilateral pelvic lymph node dissection (open)	One-time procedure that may cure prostate cancer in earlier stages. Allows for pathologic staging of disease. PSA goes to undetectable if no remaining prostate cancer.	Incontinence; impotence; bladder neck contracture. Rarely: a need for blood transfusion, nerve injury, rectal injury. Longer recovery period, 2–4% incidence of permanent incontinence. 20–40% incidence of permanent impotence. Risk of impotence and incontinence. Risk of impotence (ED) varies with nerve-sparing status and presurgical erectile function.	Yes, in setting of localized disease.	If it fails locally, external beam radiation therapy is used. If it fails in distant disease (metastases), hormones are used.
Perineal prostatectomy	One-time procedure that may cure prostate cancer in earlier stages. Allows for pathologic staging of disease. PSA goes to undetectable if no remaining prostate cancer. Avoids abdominal incision.	Lymph node dissection requires a separate procedure. Limited number of surgeons are familiar with this procedure. Risk of impotence and incontinence. Risk of impotence (ED) varies with nerve-sparing status and presurgical erectile function.	Yes, in setting of localized disease.	Same as with radical prostatectomy.

(continues)

Table 6 Initial Treatment Options for Prostate Cancer (continued)

Mode of Treatment	Advantages	Disadvantages	Curative: Yes/No	Alternative If Fails
Laparoscopic radical prostatectomy and robot-assisted radical prostatectomy	Quicker recovery; less postoperative pain; possible better visualization of pelvic anatomy. Allows for accurate staging; same advantages as RRPX. Less blood loss compared to open radical prostatectomy. Robotic vs. lap—faster OR time, easier to perform. Comparable short-term outcomes to open surgery.	Laparoscopic: A long procedure that was first pioneered by French in 1998; long-term data not available. Steep learning curve. Robotic: extremely expensive. Risk of impotence and incontinence. Risk of impotence (ED) varies with nerve-sparing status and presurgical erectile function.	Yes, if localized disease.	Locally, XRT; in distant disease, hormones are used.
External beam radiation therapy	Avoids major surgery; may cure prostate cancer in early stages. Incontinence less common than with surgery. No transfusion risk. Onset of impotence is delayed and often responds to oral therapy.	Fatigue; skin reaction in treated areas; urinary frequency and dysuria; proctitis, rectal bleeding, frequent stools, urgency; bowel function may remain abnormal; hematuria. Rare: fistula. No lymph node analysis or pathologic staging; requires treatments 5 days a week for 6 to 7 weeks; 30–50% chance of erectile dysfunction; 10–15% chance of bladder and/or rectal irritation. May have hair loss in area receiving full dose such as pubic hair. PSA doesn't go to undetectable levels.	Yes, in setting of localized disease.	Hormone treatment. Salvage prostatectomy with associated increased risk of incontinence.

Mode of Treatment	Advantages	Disadvantages	Curative: Yes/No	Alternative If Fails
Brachytherapy (interstitial seeds)	Minimally invasive; quick recovery; no transfusions.	This therapy is not for every patient (men with high grade cancer, PSA > 10, Gleason score ≥ 7, are more likely to fail). Large glands are more difficult. Urinary frequency, urgency, hematuria, rectal irritation, pain, burning, frequency and urgency with bowel movements. Chance of impotence or pain with ejaculation; 25–60% chance of impotence. No pathologic staging; urinary retention; harder to do if have had prior TURP.	Over the short term, if the prostate cancer is localized, brachytherapy appears to be curative; long-term data need to be reviewed.	Salvage prostatectomy if localized; hormones if distant disease.
HIFU (high intensity focused ultrasound) Currently FDA approved for ablation of prostate tissue	Less invasive, short hospital stay, effective in early disease.	FDA approval does not specify approved for prostate cancer, long-term efficacy data needed; lengthy procedure; ideal for monofocal well differentiated prostate cancer. Risks of urethral stricture, epdididymitis, need for TURP if large prostate; urinary retention, troubles urinating, erectile dysfunction.	Long-term data not available, recurrence rate not known, may cause scarring.	

interstitial seed therapy) are not commonly used for men with localized prostate cancer. Palliative therapies for prostate cancer include the use of hormonal therapies and radiation therapy for symptomatic bone metastases. For extensive bone metastases, systemic radionuclide therapies, such as radium 223, have proven useful in decreasing pain and skeletal related adverse events. In those individuals whose prostate cancer is refractory to hormonal therapy, chemotherapy may be an option as well as immunotherapy/vaccine therapy.

Watchful waiting

Active observation and regular monitoring of a patient without actual treatment.

Active surveillance

A form of prostate cancer therapy whereby no definitive treatment is instituted initially, but definitive therapy is instituted when predefined changes are noted.

The option of **watchful waiting/observation** or **active surveillance** can also be chosen (see Question 83). Watchful waiting involves no treatment initially. Rather, your prostate cancer is monitored with periodic PSAs and DREs and possibly X-rays. The premise of watchful waiting is that some individuals will not benefit from definitive treatment for their prostate cancer. With watchful waiting, palliative treatment (treatment designed to slow down the growth of the cancer and to treat symptoms, but not cure the cancer) is instituted for local or metastatic progression, if it occurs. Palliative therapies include: trimming of the prostate (transurethral prostatectomy) if the prostate becomes large enough that it causes trouble urinating, hormonal therapy to decrease the size and growth of the prostate cancer, and radiation therapy if symptomatic bone metastases occur.

Active surveillance differs from watchful waiting. The goal of active surveillance is to give definitive (curative) treatment to those men with prostate cancers that are likely to progress and to decrease the risk of treatment-related side effects in those men whose cancers are less likely to progress. Thus with active surveillance one also undergoes periodic PSAs and DREs, but definitive therapy is instituted when pre-defined changes are noted. The National Comprehensive Cancer Network (NCCN) has established guidelines for active surveillance. Active surveillance is better for older patients with shorter life expectancies and with lower-risk prostate cancers. Under the NCCN guidelines, active surveillance should be recommended to men with low-risk prostate cancer who have a life expectancy < 20 years (tumor stage T1–T2a, Gleason score 2–6, PSA < 10 ng/mL), very low-risk prostate cancer patients with a life expectancy up to 20 years (tumor stage T1c, Gleason score < 6, PSA less than or equal to 10, < 3 prostate biopsy cores positive, < 50% cancer in any core), and men with favorable intermediate risk prostate cancer (predominant Gleason 3 and < 50% of biopsy cores positive and no more than one NCCN intermediate risk factor) (**Table 7,** page 73). See Question 83 for more about active surveillance.

Table 7 NCCN Established Guidelines for Prostate Cancer Risk Levels

Risk Level	Clinical Stage	Gleason Score	PSA
Very Low Risk	T1C	Gleason grade group 1	≤ 10 ng/mL, < 3 biopsy cores positive, ≤ 50% in any core, PSA density <0.15 ng/mL/g
Low Risk	T1–T2a	Gleason grade group 1	< 10 ng/mL
Intermediate Risk	T2b–T2c	Gleason 3 + 4 = 7, Gleason grade group 2 Gleason 4 + 3 = 7, Gleason grade group 3	10–20 ng/mL
High Risk	T3a	Gleason 8, Gleason grade group 4 Gleason 9–10, Gleason grade group 5	> 20 ng/mL
Very High Risk	T3b–T4	Primary Gleason pattern 5, Gleason grade group 5 > 4 scores of Gleason 8–10, Gleason grade group 4 or 5	

Surgery is currently the most commonly performed treatment with the intent to cure prostate cancer. The surgical procedure is called a radical prostatectomy (see Question 52) and involves the removal of the entire prostate gland. Radical prostatectomy may be performed through an **incision** (the cutting of the skin at the beginning of surgery) that extends from the umbilicus to the pubic bone (**Figure 8**, page 74), through a perineal incision (between the scrotum and the anus) (**Figure 9**, page 75), laparoscopically (**Figure 10**, page 75), and more recently with the assistance of a robot (**Figure 11**, page 75). The choice of technique varies with the patient's body characteristics and the urologist's preference.

Open and robot-assisted radical prostatectomy have similar outcomes with respect to cancer control, recovery of urinary continence, and sexual recovery. There is less blood loss during the surgery with robot-assisted, laparoscopic, and perineal radical prostatectomy than open radical prostatectomy.

Incision

Cutting of the skin at the beginning of surgery.

Surgery is currently the most commonly performed treatment with the intent to cure prostate cancer. The surgical procedure is called a radical prostatectomy and involves the removal of the entire prostate gland.

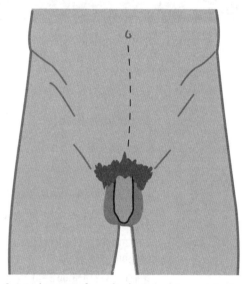

Figure 8 Surgical incision for radical retropubic prostatectomy.
A midline incision is made from the symphysis pubis to the umbilicus.

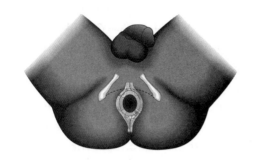

Figure 9
Radical perineal prostatectomy— incision lines.

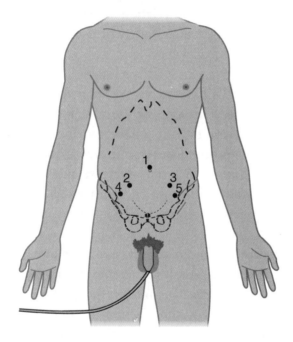

Figure 10
Trocar sites for laparoscopic radical prostatectomy.

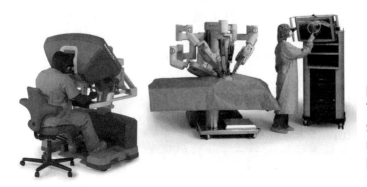

Figure 11
The da Vinci surgical system used for robotic radical prostatecomy.

Interstitial

Within an organ, such as interstitial brachytherapy, whereby radioactive seeds are placed into the prostate.

Brachytherapy

A form of radiation therapy whereby radioactive pellets are placed into the prostate.

Percutaneous

Through the skin.

Conformal EBRT

EBRT that uses CT scan images to better visualize radiation targets and normal tissues.

Cryotherapy, cryosurgery

A prostate cancer therapy in which the prostate is frozen to destroy the cancer cells.

Interstitial seed placement (**brachytherapy**) is a procedure that is minimally invasive and requires a single treatment. Similar to radical prostatectomy, it is a procedure with intent to cure. This procedure involves the **percutaneous** (through the skin) placement of radioactive seeds into the prostate (see Question 58, **Figure 12**, page 76). Depending on the prostate cancer grade and stage, Gleason grade score, and the PSA, conformal external beam radiation therapy (EBRT), in which beams of high-energy radiation are aimed at the prostate (or other target organ), may be used in addition to the interstitial seeds.

Conformal EBRT is a newer way of delivering EBRT to the prostate. Through the use of CT scanning and the improved ability to focus the maximum radiation effects on the prostate and less on the surrounding tissues, conformal EBRT may decrease side effects and improve results over those of traditional EBRT. This procedure is also performed with intent to cure.

Cryotherapy is a minimally invasive procedure in which probes are percutaneously placed into the prostate under ultrasound guidance. Liquid nitrogen, or more commonly, argon gas, is administered through the probes to "freeze" and kill the cancer cells (see Question 71). The American Urological Association's (AUA) best policy statement on cryotherapy indicates that primary cryosurgery is an option, when it is appropriate, for men who have clinically organ-confined disease of any grade with a negative metastatic evaluation (see Question 72).

Figure 12

Actual size of I-125 seeds used for brachytherapy.

Reproduced with permission from Nycomed Amersham/GE Healthcare.

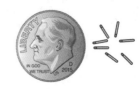

It may be more difficult in men with larger prostates (www.auanet.org). Currently, this procedure is more commonly used as a second-line procedure when an individual has not responded to EBRT. It, too, is used with intent to cure.

High-intensity focused ultrasound (HIFU) is a procedure approved more recently by the **Food and Drug Administration (FDA)** for prostate tissue ablation. The procedure is performed by inserting a probe into the rectum. The probe delivers highly focused ultrasound to the prostate. HIFU heats the prostate to temperatures of 80–100°C, which is enough to kill prostate cancer cells. The effect is limited to the prostate and does not irritate the rectal tissue. The AUA/American Society for Radiation Oncology (ASTRO) guidelines note that the use of HIFU therapy for low-risk and intermediate-risk prostate cancer is not the standard of care because comparative evidence is lacking. Furthermore, the AUA/ASTRO guidelines indicate that HIFU is not recommended in high-risk prostate cancer patients (Table 6, pages 68–71).

> **Food and Drug Administration (FDA)**
>
> Agency responsible for the approval of prescription medications in the United States.

Hormone therapy, through the use of pills, shots, both pills and shots, or bilateral orchiectomy, is a palliative approach to the treatment of prostate cancer. By removing or preventing the action of testosterone on the prostate cancer, these therapies shrink the prostate cancer and slow down its growth. However, they do not cure prostate cancer (see Question 75).

> **Hormone therapy**
>
> The manipulation of the disease's natural history and symptoms through the use of hormones.

Radiation therapy is typically used as palliative treatment for patients with pain caused by bone metastases. For men with extensive, symptomatic bone metastases, the use of a bisphosphonate, zoledronic acid (Zometa), has been approved to decrease the risk of skeletal complications in men with mCRPC. It is an intravenous

> **Radiation therapy**
>
> Use of radioactive beams or implants to kill cancer cells.

infusion that is administered every 3 to 4 weeks. Denosumab (Prolia, Xgeva), a RANK-ligand inhibitor, prevents the breakdown of bone and has been demonstrated to lower the incidence of bone fractures. It is given as a subcutaneous injection every 4 weeks. Patients need to take calcium and vitamin D with the denosumab therapy. For patients with significant pain and more extensive bone metastases, intravenous radionuclide treatments that are directed to bone metastases can be helpful. The FDA has approved several therapies, the newest one being radium 223, which has been demonstrated to not only decrease pain, but is also associated with prolonging survival by 3.6 months. Furthermore, it has less effects on the blood cell counts than previously approved radionuclide therapies.

Chemotherapy

A treatment for cancer that uses powerful medications to weaken and destroy the cancer cells.

Chemotherapy is the use of powerful drugs either to kill cancer cells or interfere with their growth. Chemotherapy drugs are good at fighting cancer because they affect mostly fast-multiplying cancer cells. Some healthy cells in the body also divide quickly, such as cells that produce hair, blood, nails, and the lining of the mouth and intestinal tract. Cells in these parts of the body can be harmed by chemotherapy. Therefore, some common side effects of chemotherapy include hair loss, low white blood cell count, nail changes, mouth and throat irritation, nausea, and vomiting.

Chemotherapy can be either injected into a vein or taken by mouth. The medicine then travels throughout the body to reach some cancer cells that may have spread beyond the prostate. Often, patients who are given hormone therapy prior to chemotherapy continue their hormone treatment through the course of their chemotherapy.

Various chemotherapy regimens are being evaluated to identify drugs that may be effective against prostate cancer. The ideal drug would be one that kills the prostate cancer, rather than just slowing down its growth. Recently, the FDA has approved the use of certain chemotherapies for men with castrate-resistant prostate cancer (those men whose prostate cancer is growing despite being on medication that prevents testosterone from being produced). Clinical trials are being performed to identify new medications and combinations of medications in hopes of identifying more effective therapies with fewer side effects (see Question 89).

Immunotherapy is the treatment of disease by inducing, enhancing, or suppressing an immune response. Vaccine therapy is a type of immune therapy which involves the injection of a chemical, an antigen, into an individual. The antigen stimulates the individual's own body to produce cells that fight off the antigen, and in doing so, kills the cancer cells. Currently, there is an FDA-approved vaccine therapy (Sipuleucel-T [Provenge]) for the treatment of asymptomatic or minimally symptomatic metastatic prostate cancer that is resistant to hormone therapy (see Question 78).

Immunotherapy
The treatment of disease by inducing, enhancing, or suppressing an immune response.

Vaccine therapy
A type of immune therapy which involved the injection of a chemical into an individual.

48. How do I decide which treatment is best for me?

Currently, the burden of medical decision-making falls on you, the patient, and it is our job as physicians to provide you with the information that will allow you to make the decision. When forced to make a difficult decision, we often rely on loved ones, close friends, and knowledgeable

TREATMENT OF PROSTATE CANCER

It is your physician's responsibility to accurately inform you of the likelihood of side effects of each of the treatment options and the remedies that are available to treat those side effects.

individuals to help us, but these people do not have to live with the effects of that decision. As you weigh the pros and cons of each of the various treatment options, it is very important that you think of how they will affect you. Now is the time to be very honest with yourself about what side effects you can and cannot tolerate. It is your physician's responsibility to accurately inform you of the likelihood of side effects of each of the treatment options and the remedies that are available to treat those side effects. When faced with a diagnosis of prostate cancer, the first impulse may be to get rid of the cancer at any cost. Unfortunately, once the prostate cancer has been treated and that worry quiets down, the side effects of the treatment can become more bothersome—so you should think seriously about them beforehand.

When counseling a patient, the first question that I typically ask is, "Can you live with your prostate inside of you over the long term?" If the answer is no, that you would be constantly worrying about whether cancer remained in the prostate if it were left in place, then a radical prostatectomy is probably best for you.

Other issues to bear in mind are the impact of incontinence and erectile dysfunction on your lifestyle. Virtually all forms of therapy can cause erectile dysfunction. If this is particularly worrisome to you, then it may be appropriate to meet with a urologist who treats erectile dysfunction to discuss the treatment options before you begin treatment for your prostate cancer. Similarly, it may be helpful to discuss the various treatments for incontinence or inability to urinate (**retention**) with your urologist or radiation oncologist before undergoing treatment. Your physician may make some treatment recommendations based on your age, medical conditions, and clinical stage of your prostate cancer. If you

Retention

Difficulty in emptying the bladder of urine; may be complete, in which one is unable to void, or partial, in which urine is left in the bladder after voiding.

have questions as to why certain recommendations are being made, now is the time to ask them. Remember, no question is stupid. Your physician wants you to feel comfortable with your decision and will help you find the information that you need. There are also organizations that can provide you with information regarding treatment and side effects (see **Appendix**).

In an effort to help determine which therapies have the best chance of curing you of your prostate cancer, researchers have stratified prostate cancer into several risk levels for disease progression (see Table 7, page 73). The treatment recommendations vary with the risk.

Low-risk patients usually can be treated with active surveillance; however, some also do well with a single therapy such as radical prostatectomy, external beam radiation therapy, or interstitial seed therapy. High-risk patients are more likely to experience a treatment failure and combination therapy such as external beam therapy and hormonal therapy is often recommended.

There are several biomarkers that may be used to help predict the "aggressiveness" of the prostate cancer (see Table 1, page 10). Not all of these biomarkers' tests are currently covered by insurance companies. Some of these biomarker tests include:

- **SCHLAP1**—This test may help predict the likelihood of the prostate cancer spreading (metastasizing). High SCHLAP1 has been associated with a higher risk of biochemical recurrence, metastases, and death from prostate cancer.
- **Decipher**—This is a gene-based test used for patients with a history of a positive prostate biopsy and is also used in men who have undergone a radical

SCHLAP1

Potential biomarker for the determination of risk of prostate cancer metastatic progression.

Decipher

22 gene based test that predicts the likelihood of high-grade prostate cancer and metastatic disease after radical prostatectomy.

prostatectomy. This test predicts the likelihood of (1) the presence of high-grade (Gleason 4 or 5) prostate cancer and (2) the risk of metastases and prostate cancer related death in men with prostate cancer who have undergone radical prostatectomy.

- ELAVL—A test that measures an RNA binding protein that may play a role in the progression of prostate cancer. It can predict the aggressiveness of the prostate cancer and the risk of recurrence of the prostate cancer after treatment.

Oncotype Dx

Gene based assay (12 genes)—a score is developed, the GPS, genomic prostate score, which assesses likelihood of favorable pathology.

Prolaris

Uses a score based on level of expression of mRNA of 31 cell cycle progression genes and 15 housekeeping genes.

- **OncotypeDx**—A complex genetic-based test to further stratify low and low-intermediate risk prostate cancer (Gleason score 6 or low volume Gleason 3 + 4). This test uses 12 cancer-related genes and 5 reference genes to provide a score, the GPS (genomic prostate score). This test is helpful in determining which men are suitable for active surveillance.

- **Prolaris**—A genetic test that looks at 31 genes that are involved in the growth of cells compared to 15 other genes and provides a "cell cycle progression" score that may be helpful in determining the need for treatment versus active surveillance.

49. Some of my good friends have prostate cancer and have undergone various treatments with good results. Should I have what they had?

It is often helpful to discuss with your friends how they made their final treatment decisions. They may be able to help you develop a list of questions and concerns to address with your doctor(s). Remember, however, that everyone is different and what may be appropriate for your friend may not be appropriate for you. Your Gleason score, PSA, volume of cancer, and overall health status may be different from those of your friends. Your friend may not be able to cope with his prostate remaining in place and may desire a radical prostatectomy at all costs, whereas you may be very concerned about urinary incontinence, and this concern may drive your decision making. Thus, the ultimate decision should be yours.

50. How do I select my urologist, radiation oncologist, and/or oncologist?

Cliff's comment:

My first urologist, the individual who performed my prostate biopsies, thoroughly explained the three options of treatment to me: radiation, seeds, or radical prostatectomy. However, his presentation was abrupt, showed no compassion, and sounded like a recited speech. I had done some reading on prostate cancer and asked him some questions. When I tried to discuss his qualifications and his success with preserving erectile function, his response was that his results are as good as any other doctors in the area and that if I wanted better, I should go to Johns Hopkins. Then he bluntly said that I should just assume that I would be impotent after the surgery—he WASN'T FOR ME! The urologist that I ultimately chose to perform my surgery was patient, sympathetic to my situation and feelings, and discussed with me the issue of potency and his success rates with the nerve-sparing radical prostatectomy. He indicated that given my Gleason score, PSA, and biopsy results, he would try to spare one set of nerves in the hope of preserving my erectile function. HE WAS THE ONE FOR ME!

As discussed in Question 46, it is common for prostate cancer patients to be treated by a multidisciplinary team of physicians and other healthcare providers. This team system, in which each clinician provides care in his or her area of medical expertise, has become a standard approach in modern cancer treatment.

When choosing a urologist for your prostate biopsies (and subsequent management if the biopsies are positive), you should consider a urologist who deals with prostate cancer on a regular basis.

Complication

An undesirable result of a treatment, surgery, or medication.

If your primary care provider is performing your prostate cancer screening and detects an abnormality in your PSA and/or rectal examination, he or she may refer you to a urologist or to a urology practice for further evaluation. When choosing a urologist for your prostate biopsies (and subsequent management if the biopsies are positive), you should consider a urologist who deals with prostate cancer on a regular basis. Several issues should be considered when you select a physician:

Competence. You want a capable doctor who is knowledgeable and can apply that knowledge.

Technical skills. If you are planning to have prostate cancer surgery, you want to select an individual who performs a lot of radical prostatectomies. The urologist should know his or her own complication rate (a **complication** is an undesirable result of a treatment) and success rate and should feel comfortable discussing these with you. The old dictum "practice makes perfect" holds true to some extent.

Compassion. Cancer is a scary word and disease no matter how you look at it. You want a physician who understands this and is willing to take the time to help you make your management decision so that you will feel comfortable with your decision.

Approachability. As you go through the decision-making process, you want to be able to ask questions of your physician and have these questions answered in a timely manner. Delays in diagnosis and treatment only add to your anxiety.

Communication. You should expect that the team of physicians and others who are managing your case will communicate appropriately and effectively with one another as well as directly with you.

The same concepts apply in your choice of an **oncologist** (a medical specialist who is trained to evaluate and treat cancer) or radiation oncologist (a physician who treats cancer through the use of radiation therapy). Friends who have prostate cancer may also be able to assist you with the identification of a urologist, oncologist, or radiation oncologist who specializes in the treatment of prostate cancer.

Oncologist

A medical specialist who is trained to evaluate and treat cancer.

51. Should I get a second opinion?

Cliff's comment:

I think a second opinion is imperative if you have any doubt in your mind. Remember, it is your life and you want the best advice.

The decision of how best to treat your prostate cancer is a big one. You may feel very comfortable with the information that you have been given by your urologist/radiation oncologist/oncologist and you may be comfortable making an educated decision. If you do not feel that you have received enough information or you are concerned about the treatment recommendations that your urologist/radiation oncologist/oncologist is making, then it is appropriate to seek a second opinion. With all forms of therapy, it is important to ensure that those at the location where you will be receiving treatment are experienced with the form of therapy that you are selecting. It is not unreasonable to ask the urologist or radiation oncologist/oncologist what his or her or the institution's success, failure, and complication rates are. It is easy for the doctor to quote the results of large studies that show a course of treatment to be effective and safe, but what is important to you are the results of your local team. If you are concerned because of a lack of information regarding these results, it may also be appropriate to seek a second opinion. Some patients are afraid to seek second opinions because they are worried that their doctor will be offended, but most physicians understand the difficult decisions that you have to make and want you to feel as comfortable as you can with your decision. In fact, many help arrange for copies of your pathology reports, clinic notes, lab tests, and X-ray results to be forwarded to the doctor you are seeing for a second opinion.

Radical prostatectomy is the surgical procedure whereby the entire prostate is removed, as well as the seminal vesicles, the section of the urethra that passes through the prostate, the ends of the vas deferens, and a portion of the bladder neck.

Catheter

A hollow tube that allows for fluid drainage from or injection into an area.

52. What is a radical prostatectomy? What are the risks and complications of radical prostatectomy?

Radical prostatectomy is the surgical procedure whereby the entire prostate is removed, as well as the seminal vesicles, the section of the urethra that passes through the prostate, the ends of the vas deferens, and a portion of the bladder neck. After the prostate and surrounding structures are removed, the bladder is then reattached to the remaining urethra. A **catheter**, which is a hollow tube, is placed through the penis into the bladder before the stitches that attach the bladder to the urethra are tied down. The catheter allows urine to drain while the bladder and urethra heal together. Because some mild bleeding, lymph drainage, and urine drainage may occur, a small drain may be placed through the skin of the abdomen into the pelvis. This drain is removed when the fluid output decreases. At the time of radical prostatectomy, depending on the approach used, the pelvic lymph nodes, which are a common location of prostate cancer metastases, may also be removed (see Question 44). A radical prostatectomy may be performed via three different approaches. In the open retropubic approach, an incision is made that extends from the umbilicus (belly button) to the symphysis pubis (pubic bone) (Figure 8, page 74). The radical prostatectomy may also be performed laparoscopically through several small incisions made in various locations in the abdomen (Figures 8 and 10, pages 74–75), or through a perineal approach, with the incision being made in the area between the scrotum and the anus (Figure 9, page 75). More recently, the radical prostatectomy may be performed with the use of a robot, robot-assisted radical prostatectomy, which is similar to laparoscopic surgery in that it is less invasive than open surgery (Figure 11, page 75).

Radical prostatectomy differs from a TURP and an open suprapubic prostatectomy in that the entire prostate is removed in a radical prostatectomy. Therefore, unlike TURP and open suprapubic prostatectomy, the PSA should decrease to an undetectable level within a month or so after the procedure if no prostate cancer cells are present.

The decision as to what approach will be used for a radical prostatectomy depends on your urologist's preference and skills, your body characteristics, and whether a pelvic lymph node dissection is planned.

An advantage of the retropubic approach is that it allows for easy access to the pelvic lymph nodes so that a pelvic lymph node dissection can be performed easily at the same time. In addition, the blood vessels and nerves that control your potency are visualized easily. A disadvantage of this procedure is the abdominal incision, which may lead to a longer recovery time and increased

Perineal prostatectomy

Removal of the entire prostate, seminal vesicles, and part of the vas deferens through an incision made in the perineum.

Laparoscopic radical prostatectomy

Removal of the entire prostate, seminal vesicles, and part of the vas deferens via the laparoscope.

Laparoscopic radical prostatectomy is a procedure that has the advantages of the retropubic approach, but because there are several small abdominal incisions as opposed to the longer midline incision, the discomfort is less and the recovery is quicker with this approach.

discomfort and a higher blood loss compared to laparoscopic and robot-assisted radical prostatectomy.

The **perineal prostatectomy** does not involve an abdominal incision and is reported to be less uncomfortable and the recovery period shorter. The perineal approach allows for good visualization of the outlet of the bladder and the urethra for sewing the two together; however, the nerves that control potency are not seen as easily as with the retropubic approach. Another disadvantage of this procedure is that it does not allow for removal of the pelvic lymph nodes through the perineal incision and would require an additional incision for the pelvic lymph node dissection. This procedure is best suited for overweight men, for whom the retropubic approach is more difficult.

Laparoscopic radical prostatectomy is a procedure that has the advantages of the retropubic approach, but because there are several small abdominal incisions as opposed to the longer midline incision, the discomfort is less and the recovery is quicker with this approach. The disadvantage of this procedure is that it requires a surgeon skilled in **laparoscopy** (surgery performed through small incisions with visualization provided by a small telescope instrument and fine instruments that fit through the small incisions), and currently appears to be taking longer to perform than a robot-assisted radical prostatectomy. The outcomes of laparoscopic prostatectomy, i.e., urinary incontinence, erectile function, and positive margin (cancer cells at the edge of the specimen) rates are similar to open surgery.

Robot-assisted radical prostatectomy is the newest form of minimally invasive surgery for prostate cancer. The procedure is performed using a 3- or 4-armed robot.

The robot is controlled by the surgeon, who sits at a specialized desk and controls movement of the robot's arms. Advantages of robot-assisted prostatectomy are its ease of use compared to laparoscopy and the surgery tends to be quicker as compared to laparoscopy. In addition, the arms of the robot have movements similar to a human arm/hand/wrist, but the tremors that may be present with human movements are controlled. The robotic arms have a greater range of motion than a human arm. Also, the blood loss associated with robot-assisted radical prostatectomy is lower than with open radical prostatectomy. A disadvantage of the robot is the expense of the robot; not all hospitals can afford to purchase a robot. The outcomes (cancer control, continence, and sexual recovery) with the robot are similar to those of laparoscopic and open radical prostatectomy (Figure 10, page 75).

All surgical procedures have risks, and the common ones are infection, bleeding, pain, and anesthetic complications. Larger surgical procedures, which involve lengthier operative times and decreased postoperative mobility, have the risk of blood clots in the legs (deep venous thrombosis), pulmonary embolus, pneumonia, and stress-related stomach ulcers. Complications of radical prostatectomy include **hernia** (a weakening in the muscle that leads to a bulge), significant bleeding requiring blood transfusion, infection, anesthetic-related complications, impotence, urinary incontinence, bladder neck contracture, lymphocele (see lymphocele under risks of lymph node dissection, Question 44), deep venous thrombosis, rectal injury, and death.

Bleeding

There are several large blood vessels in the pelvis and around the prostate, including the dorsal vein, which lies on top of the prostate. In order to remove the prostate,

TREATMENT OF PROSTATE CANCER

Laparoscopy

A surgical procedure in which a fiber-optic instrument is inserted through the abdominal wall to view the organs in the abdomen or to permit a surgical procedure.

Robot-assisted radical prostatectomy

A radical prostatectomy performed with the assistance of a robot.

Hernia

A weakening in the muscle that leads to a bulge, often in the groin.

this large vein is often tied off and cut, which could cause significant and rapid bleeding. In most cases, the blood loss is less than one pint (**unit**) of blood, but in about 5% to 10% of cases, a blood transfusion is required. The amount of blood loss tends to be lower with both laparoscopic and robot-assisted radical prostatectomies compared to open radical retropubic prostatectomy.

Unit

Term referring to a pint of blood.

Infection

Several different types of infections can occur with this surgery. A skin infection (cellulitis) may occur at the incision, an abscess (a collection of pus) may occur under the skin or deep in the pelvis, or a urinary tract infection may occur. A skin infection at the incision typically presents with redness, swelling, tenderness, and occasionally, drainage at the incision. In the absence of pus, this usually can be treated successfully with oral antibiotics; rarely, intravenous antibiotics are indicated.

Abscesses are collections of pus and may occur just under the skin or deeper in the pelvis and require drainage.

More superficial abscesses can be treated by opening the incision, draining the pus, and packing the wound with sterile gauze; the packing is continued until the area heals. If the abscess is in the pelvis, it can often be treated by placing a drain through the skin into the abscess and draining the pus. This is often done under X-ray guidance by an interventional radiologist.

Urinary tract infections result from the catheter, which drains the bladder during the healing process. The risk of a urinary tract infection increases with the number of days that the catheter is in place. Because most urologists leave the catheter in for 1 to 2 weeks after the surgery, your urologist may have you drop a urine sample off at the lab 2 to 3 days before the catheter is removed so that they can detect whether any bacteria are present and if so, treat them to prevent an infection after the catheter has been removed or prescribe antibiotics at the time of the catheter removal. Signs of a urinary tract infection include frequent urination, urgency and discomfort with urination, and sometimes a low-grade fever.

Anesthetic Complications

Most patients undergo **general anesthesia** (anesthesia involving total loss of consciousness) for their radical prostatectomy; however, the procedure may be performed under spinal anesthesia. **Epidural anesthesia** may be used to improve postoperative pain control and decrease intra-operative anesthetic requirements. The most commonly encountered side effects of general anesthesia are scratchy throat, nausea, and vomiting, but significant anesthetic complications are rare. With epidural catheters, potential side effects include lowering of the blood pressure and muscle blocks, which may affect movement of a leg. With less invasive procedures, such as robot-assisted radical prostatectomy, there appears to be less pain.

Impotence

Impotence, or **erectile dysfunction**, is unfortunately a commonly identified risk of radical prostatectomy via any technique. The risk of postoperative erectile dysfunction increases with increased age at the time of the surgery. The nerves that supply the penis and that are involved in the erectile process lie along each side of the prostate and the urethra. They may be taken deliberately by the surgeon (non–nerve-sparing radical prostatectomy), or they may be injured permanently or transiently. When the surgeon tries to avoid injury to the nerves, this is called a nerve-sparing prostatectomy. The decision to try to spare one or both nerve bundles varies with

General anesthesia

Anesthesia which involves total loss of consciousness.

Epidural anesthesia

A special type of anesthesia whereby pain medications are placed through a catheter in the back, into the fluid that surrounds the spinal cord.

The most commonly encountered side effects of general anesthesia are scratchy throat, nausea, and vomiting, but significant anesthetic complications are rare.

Erectile dysfunction

The inability to achieve and/or maintain an erection satisfactory for the completion of sexual performance.

your surgeon's expertise, your Gleason score, your PSA level, and the volume (amount) of tumor on the biopsies. The incidence of postoperative erectile dysfunction may be as low as 25% in men younger than 60 who undergo bilateral nerve-sparing radical prostatectomy, or it may be as high as 62% in men older than 70 who undergo unilateral nerve-sparing radical prostatectomy. Many factors can affect your erectile function after surgery, including your erectile function before surgery, your age, your pathological tumor stage, and the extent of preservation of the nerves. Erectile dysfunction after radical prostatectomy may resolve over the first year or two after surgery. During that time, and if the trouble persists, you may seek treatment for it (see Question 91). Some studies have demonstrated that recovery of erectile function may be improved by using medical therapies early after radical prostatectomy until normal erectile function returns (penile rehabilitation). After a radical prostatectomy, you have no ejaculate because the sources of the fluid are either removed (prostate and seminal vesicles) or tied off (the vas deferens). However, you may still experience climax (reach an orgasm).

Many factors can affect your erectile function after surgery, including your erectile function before surgery, your age, your pathological tumor stage, and the extent of preservation of the nerves.

Urinary Incontinence

Urinary incontinence is another risk of radical prostatectomy.

Urinary incontinence

The unintentional loss of urine.

Cliff's comment:

I feared this risk the most. I remember getting the diapers and pads the day that I had my catheter removed—my God, I thought, I am 60 years old and I'm going to be wearing diapers. Needless to say, my wife had no sympathy when I moaned about the possibility of having to wear a pad. I was lucky, however; I had two small "spills" at night and that was it for my incontinence. I discarded all of those diapers and pads within a week.

Incontinence may vary from none to persistent incontinence, such that every time you move you leak urine. The more common type of incontinence is stress-related incontinence, which is leakage that occurs when you increase the pressure in your abdomen, such as when you bear down, pick up something heavy, laugh, or cough. The incidence of incontinence varies from 1% to 58%, and one of the reasons for the wide range in the reported incidence of incontinence is that the definition of incontinence varies. If one considers any leakage that occurs to be incontinence, then the incidence would be higher than if incontinence were defined as leakage sufficient to change a pad a day. As with erectile dysfunction, incontinence may improve or resolve over time. Risks for incontinence after surgery include prior pelvic irradiation and older age. Many options are available for the treatment of urinary incontinence after radical prostatectomy (see Question 92).

Bladder Neck Contracture

A **bladder neck contracture** is scar tissue that develops in the area where the bladder and urethra are sewn together. This problem occurs in about 1 in every 20 to 30 prostatectomies. The signs and symptoms of a bladder neck contracture include decreased force of stream and straining (pushing) to urinate. The bladder neck contracture is identified during an office cystoscopy, in which a **cystoscope**, a telescope-like instrument, is passed through the urethra up to the bladder neck and the narrowed area is visualized. If the opening is very small, a small wire can be passed through it and the area dilated (stretched open) using some metal or plastic dilators in the office. Before the procedure, the urethra is numbed with lidocaine jelly to decrease discomfort. Usually, once the bladder neck is dilated, it remains open; however, in a small number of men, a repeat

Bladder neck contracture

Scar tissue at the bladder neck that causes narrowing.

Cystoscope

A telescope-like instrument that allows one to examine the urethra and inside of the bladder.

dilation or an incision into the scar under anesthesia is needed. A complication of treatment for bladder neck contracture is urinary incontinence.

Deep Venous Thrombosis

A **deep venous thrombosis** (**DVT**) is a blood clot that develops in the veins in the leg or the pelvis. People with cancer and those who are sedentary are at increased risk for such blood clots. During surgery and your initial postoperative period, you are not moving around much and are at increased risk for forming blood clots. Thromboembolic (TED) hose and Venodynes (pneumatic sequential stockings that inflate and deflate to keep blood flowing) are often used during this period to decrease the risk of forming such blood clots. Some surgeons choose subcutaneous low molecular weight heparin to prevent DVTs. DVTs may cause swelling of the leg, which often resolves when the blood clot dissolves.

A more serious risk posed by a DVT is that a piece of the clot could break off and travel to the heart and lungs; this is called a pulmonary embolus. A pulmonary embolus can be life threatening if the fragment is large enough to block off blood flow to the lung. DVTs may occur after you are discharged from the hospital. Thus, if you note acute swelling and/or pain in your lower leg(s), you should contact your doctor.

Rectal Injury

The incidence of rectal injury during a radical prostatectomy is less than 2%. There is a slightly higher risk of rectal injury with the perineal approach (1.73%) than with the retropubic approach (0.68%). In most cases, if the injury is small and there is no stool visible, then the area can be closed and should heal. For large injuries and if there is a significant amount of stool in the bowel, a temporary **colostomy** (the bowel is brought to the skin to drain the stool into a bag) is made to decrease the chances of stool leakage and abscess formation; the colostomy can be removed later.

Colostomy

A surgical opening between the colon (large intestine) and the skin that allows stool to drain into a collecting bag.

Miscellaneous Complications Related to the Radical Prostatectomy

The retropubic prostatectomy has a higher risk of cardiovascular, respiratory, and other medically related complications, primarily **gastrointestinal** (i.e., related to the digestive system or intestines), such as the slow return of bowel function, than the perineal approach. The perineal approach has a higher risk of miscellaneous surgical complications, such as rectal injury and postoperative infections. The perineal approach may also be associated with an increased risk of incontinence of stool. The incidence of complications and **mortality** (death) increases with patient age at the time of surgery.

Gastrointestinal

Related to the digestive system and/or the intestines.

Mortality

Death related to disease or treatment.

Death

The mortality rate associated with radical prostatectomy is less than 0.1%.

53. What is a nerve-sparing radical prostatectomy?

The nerves responsible for erectile function run along each side of the prostate and along each side of the urethra before passing out of the pelvis into the penis. These nerves travel along with blood vessels, and the group is called the "neurovascular bundle," which lies outside of the prostate capsule. These nerves are not responsible for control of urine—only erectile function. During a **nerve-sparing prostatectomy**, the urologist attempts to dissect (push aside) the neurovascular

Nerve-sparing

With regard to prostate cancer, it is the attempt to avoid damaging or removing the nerves that lie on either side of the prostate gland that are in part responsible for normal erections. Injury to the nerves can cause erectile dysfunction.

bundle from the prostate and the urethra. The surgeon may perform a bilateral nerve-sparing radical prostatectomy, in which the neurovascular bundle on each side is spared, or a unilateral nerve-sparing prostatectomy, in which one neurovascular bundle is removed with the prostate. The decision of whether or not to perform a nerve-sparing radical prostatectomy depends on many issues, one of which is your erectile function. If you already have erectile dysfunction, then sparing the nerves is not an issue. Other considerations include the amount of tumor present in your biopsy specimen, the location of the tumor (whether it is in both sides of the prostate), and the Gleason score. Remember that a radical prostatectomy is a cancer operation, and the goal of the procedure is to try to remove all of the cancer. Therefore, if you are at high risk for having cancer at the edge of the prostate, it is better to remove the neurovascular bundle(s) and surrounding tissue on that side in hopes of removing all of the cancer. A bilateral nerve-sparing radical prostatectomy does not guarantee that you will have normal erectile function after the surgery. You should consider this fact and decide before surgery how much of an impact postoperative erectile dysfunction would have on your life.

54. Who is a candidate for radical prostatectomy?

The ideal candidate for a radical prostatectomy is a man who is believed to have prostate cancer that is confined to the prostate gland, is healthy enough to withstand the general anesthesia and the surgical procedure, and is expected to live for at least an additional 7 to 10 years so that he will benefit from the surgery. The AUA/ASTRO guidelines indicate that radical prostatectomy (includes open, perineal, laparoscopic, and

The ideal candidate for a radical prostatectomy is a man who is believed to have prostate cancer that is confined to the prostate gland, is healthy enough to withstand the general anesthesia and the surgical procedure, and is expected to live for at least an additional 7 to 10 years so that he will benefit from the surgery.

robotic) is considered a standard treatment option for men with intermediate-risk prostate cancer as well as those with high-risk prostate cancer. It is difficult to determine who really has organ-confined disease, or cancer that is apparently confined to the prostate. Tables may help estimate the risks of having a tumor outside of the prostate, but these are only part of the decision-making process (Table 5, pages 48–52). Approximately 20% to 60% of men undergoing radical prostatectomy have a higher stage of prostate cancer when the pathologist reviews the surgical specimen.

Just because you are a candidate for a radical prostatectomy does not mean that this is the best form of treatment for you. You must look carefully at your lifestyle, the risks of the surgery, and what is most important to you regarding your quality of life before making a decision. If, for example, the possibility of urinary incontinence would be devastating to you, then maybe surgery is not the best therapy for you. On the other hand, if the idea of leaving your prostate in place will constantly worry you, then perhaps surgery is best for you.

55. How does one prepare for radical prostatectomy?

Cliff's comment:

As you prepare for surgery and try to optimize your physical health by eating right, resting, and getting exercise, it is also important to make sure that you are able to cope mentally with all of the stress caused by the diagnosis and treatment of a cancer. I knew I was anxious about my surgery, but I was never able to correlate the significance of that until after the surgery, when I realized that I had increased the dose of my blood pressure medications significantly in the month before surgery. If you find that you are having trouble emotionally preparing for surgery, talk with your doctor, family, or friends. They may be able to help alleviate your anxieties or refer you to another individual, such as a therapist, psychologist, or psychiatrist.

In preparation for surgery, you will undergo a history and physical examination, some blood tests, and often a chest X-ray study and electrocardiogram. These assessments are performed to make sure that you are healthy enough for surgery and to rule out any medical problems that may increase your risk of complications after surgery. You should eat a healthy diet and continue to exercise before the surgery. Starting about 10 days before surgery, you should not take any medications that contain aspirin or nonsteroidal anti-inflammatory drugs, such as ibuprofen, because they might increase your risk of bleeding during the surgery. Many over-the-counter medications contain one of these, and if you are unsure about whether yours does, you should consult a pharmacist. If you were prescribed aspirin because of heart disease, then you should speak to your primary care doctor or heart doctor before stopping the aspirin.

Bowel preparation

Cleansing (and sterilization) of the intestines before abdominal surgery.

Your urologist may give you a **bowel preparation** to clean out the lower intestines. This may involve laxatives and/or an enema to clean out your bowels. You will also probably be asked to have a clear liquid diet the day before surgery and nothing to eat after midnight prior to the surgery.

56. What is the hospital course like?

Cliff's comment:

I envisioned staying in the hospital 2 to 3 days after my surgery, staying locally until the catheter was removed, and then returning home. Although my biggest fear, that of not waking up after the surgery, did not occur, I did have a rocky postoperative course and remained in the hospital for about two weeks and had the catheter in place longer. I found the catheter to be most annoying initially. I had a visiting nurse who taught me how to use the drainage bags, and I got used to the catheter, but I must admit, the day of the catheter removal was a glorious day—the ability to urinate again on my own and to control urination again felt wonderful. Thank God for those small pleasures!

Typically, you are admitted to the hospital the day of your surgery, and you usually stay in the hospital 1 to 2 nights (inpatient), including the night of your surgery for the radical retropubic prostatectomy. Men undergoing laparoscopic and robot-assisted radical prostatectomies may go home as soon as the day after surgery and tend to be fully recovered more quickly than those who undergo the traditional radical retropubic prostatectomy. Most men go from the recovery room to a regular hospital room, with very few needing a bed in the intensive care unit (ICU).

An epidural catheter, which is a small catheter placed through the lower back into the space around the spinal cord at the time of your surgery, may be used for postoperative pain control with open surgery. Pain medications can be given through the catheter to numb the nerves so that you do not feel pain. Another way to control postoperative pain is with a patient-controlled analgesia pump, which is an intravenous form of pain medication controlled by a small button that you press when you want pain medication. With laparoscopic and robot-assisted laparoscopic radical prostatectomy, these pain therapies are rarely needed, and most men are able to have their pain managed with oral pain medications. Once you are tolerating liquids, oral pain medications may be used; some physicians use narcotics, like acetaminophen (Tylenol) with codeine or oxycodone with

Typically, you are admitted to the hospital the day of your surgery, and you usually stay in the hospital 1 to 2 nights (inpatient), including the night of your surgery for the radical retropubic prostatectomy.

acetaminophen (Percocet), whereas others use strong anti-inflammatories like ketorolac tromethamine (Toradol), which doesn't slow down your bowel function. A small drain may be left in place that is connected to a bulb, which allows urine and lymph fluid to be drained out of the pelvis. The drain is removed at the bedside or during office visit when the output is minimal.

The nurses will teach you how to use the urinary drainage bags and will assist you with getting into and out of bed. You will go home when you are comfortable while taking oral pain medications and your bowels are working. You will be discharged with a **Foley catheter**, which drains the urine and will be in place 7 days to 2 weeks to allow the area where the bladder has been reattached to the urethra to heal. At home, you can resume your regular diet and slowly increase your activity level. Depending on the approach used, your full recovery may take up to one month.

After your catheter has been removed, you will be taught pelvic muscle strengthening exercises, which will help you control your urine. Most individuals regain nearly all or full control of their urine around one month after the catheter is removed. Your PSA level will be checked 4 to 6 weeks after surgery to make sure that it has decreased to an undetectable level and periodically thereafter.

57. What is the success rate of radical prostatectomy (includes open, perineal, laparoscopic, and robotic)?

Cliff's comment:

It has been 2½ years since my radical prostatectomy, and I feel great. I am doing all of the things that I had done before

Foley catheter

A latex or silicone catheter that drains urine from the bladder.

the surgery and more. So far, my PSA has remained unde-tectable, and it is very reassuring to hear this at my urology clinic visits.

In general, more than 70% of properly selected cases (i.e., men who are believed to have prostate cancer that is clinically confined to the prostate) remain free of tumor for more than 7 to 10 years. If one has a T2 tumor (see Question 42), the probability of remaining free from PSA elevation can be as high as 90% if there were no **positive margins** (tumor at the edge of the specimen). However, it is hard to predict before surgery who is the best candidate for surgery because 30% to 40% of patients are diagnosed with a higher stage or grade of cancer when the surgical specimen is reviewed by the pathologist. Positive surgical margins are found in 14% to 41% of men undergoing radical prostatectomy, and in those men with positive margins, there is an almost 50% chance that the PSA will increase within 5 years after surgery. This varies with the amount of tumor at the margin and the location of the positive margin. Your urologist would discuss whether additional ther-apy is indicated if the margin is positive. Men with negative margins have only an 18% chance of the PSA rising at 5 years after surgery. Initially after surgery, you will have your PSA level checked every 3 months. Depending on the lab that your physician uses, a PSA level < 0.1 ng/mL or a PSA level < 0.02 ng/mL may be reported as undetectable. The numbers vary because the **sensitivity** in PSA testing varies from lab to lab. If the PSA remains undetectable after 1 year, then your urolo-gist may order PSA testing every 6 months for about 1 year, after which you will continue with yearly PSA tests. Depending on your pathology report and your urologist's preference, you may also have a DRE at the time of your PSA.

TREATMENT OF PROSTATE CANCER

Positive margin

The presence of cancer cells at the cut edge of tissue removed during surgery. A posi-tive margin indi-cates that there may be cancer cells remaining in the body.

Sensitivity

The probability that a diagnostic test can correctly identify the presence of a partic-ular disease.

Cliff's comment:

The first PSA test after surgery is the most suspenseful. Even though your urologist may tell you that your pathology specimen from surgery looks good and that there are no cancer cells at the margins (the edges of the tissue), you are still anxious to hear what the PSA is. You want it to be undetectable—you want it to indicate that the cancer has been "caught" and removed. You get your blood drawn and then you wait to meet with your urologist or for the phone call regarding your results. I remember how happy I felt when I got my first PSA report after the surgery. Now, 2 ½ years later, I am still slightly anxious when I have my PSA drawn, although as each year goes by the anxiety is decreasing. With each good PSA result, I start to believe that "they've gotten it all." I realize that it will be an additional seven more years before I can technically say I am cured, but each year that goes by that I am healthy and the PSA remains undetectable is another year enjoyed and another year closer to that goal.

58. What is brachytherapy/interstitial seed therapy? What are the side effects and complications of interstitial seeds or brachytherapy?

Brachytherapy derives from the Greek word "brachy," which means "near to." Brachytherapy is a technique in which either permanent radioactive seeds or temporary needles are placed directly into the prostate gland (Figure 12, page 76 and **Figure 13**, page 103). This form of therapy started in the early 1900s and then had a resurgence in the 1970s but was abandoned because of difficulties with accurate seed placement. With the development of transrectal ultrasound (TRUS), the use of C-arm fluoroscopy, and more recently, the use of three-dimensional (3D) computerized treatment planning and postoperative CT-based dosimetry, the procedure has become technically easier and more precise.

Two radioactive agents can be used for permanent seed placement, palladium 103 and iodine 125, and both are effective in the treatment of prostate cancer. A third agent, iridium 192, is used for temporary placement and is removed after 24 to 72 hours. Palladium gives a higher initial dose of radiation when it is placed, and some people

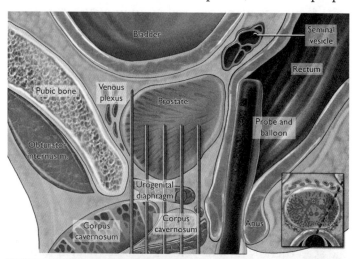

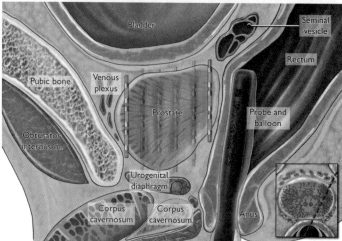

Figure 13 Template used to guide interstitial seed placement.
Courtesy of Varian Medical Systems.

think that it may be more helpful in high-grade, fast-growing tumors. Palladium tends to be used for tumors with a Gleason score of at least 7, and iodine is used for tumors with a Gleason score of 6 or less. Before the seeds are placed, either a TRUS or a CT scan of the prostate is performed to assess the prostate volume. This helps determine needle placement and seed positioning within the needle. Typically, the target volume includes the original prostate volume plus 2-mm margins laterally and anterior to the prostate gland, as well as additional 5-mm margins at the top and bottom of the prostate. This measurement is done to try to ensure that the prostatic capsule is included in the treatment. No additional margins are added posteriorly to prevent injury to the rectum. It is also important to limit the dose received by the urethra to prevent urethral irritation. Typically, a dose of 144 Gy is given for iodine 125, and 125 Gy is given for palladium 103. Iodine 125 has a half-life of 60 days, whereas palladium has a half-life of only 17 days.

The most commonly encountered side effects of interstitial seed therapy include voiding troubles related to bladder outlet obstruction, urinary incontinence, and rectal ulceration and bleeding. In addition, in some patients a benign increase in the PSA may occur after interstitial seed therapy, this is referred to as a PSA bounce or blip. Urinary symptoms occur earlier with palladium because it releases high energy earlier than iodine. Individuals may develop urinary **frequency** (frequent urination), **dysuria**, or urinary retention. Urinary symptoms, if they are not associated with urinary retention, are often treated with nonsteroidal anti-inflammatories and an **alpha-blocker**, such as doxazosin (Cardura), terazosin (Hytrin), alfuzosin (Uroxatral), silodosin (Rapaflo), and tamsulosin (Flomax), and often resolve over 1 to 4 months, but may persist for 12 to 18 months.

Frequency

A term used to describe the need to urinate often.

Dysuria

Painful urination.

Alpha blocker

An alpha adrenergic receptor blocker used to treat benign prostatic enlargement.

Bladder Outlet Obstruction

Trouble urinating after interstitial seed therapy occurs in 7% to 25% of cases, possibly as a result of blood clots in the bladder or swelling of the prostate. About 10% of men will experience acute urinary retention, the inability to urinate on their own, requiring temporary placement of a Foley catheter. If the cause is blood clots, then the clots are washed out of the bladder and a Foley catheter may be left in place for a few days. If the problems with voiding are believed to be caused by prostate swelling, then a catheter may be left in place for a short period of time, and your doctor may want you to try some medications, including an alpha-blocker, such as doxasin (Cardura), terazosin (Hytrin), tamsulosin (Flomax), silodosin (Rapaflo), alfuzosin (Rapaflo), or an anti-inflammatory (e.g., ibuprofen). If you are not able to void for awhile, then a suprapubic tube or clean intermittent **catheterization** may be easier for you. A suprapubic tube is a catheter that is placed through the skin of the lower abdomen into the bladder to drain the urine. It remains in place until you can urinate on your own. It has the advantages of being able to be changed on a monthly basis in your urologist's office, and it does not cause urethral irritation like a Foley catheter.

Clean intermittent catheterization involves placing a catheter through the penis into the bladder to drain the bladder on a regular schedule (usually every 4 to 6 hours) throughout the day. The advantages of clean intermittent catheterization are that it allows you to know when you are able to void on your own, it minimizes bladder and urethral irritation, and it has less risk of infections and bladder stones over the long term. Although it is discouraging to be unable to urinate after the procedure, it is important to allow time to pass and see whether the problem will resolve. A TURP should be delayed to

Catheterization

The insertion of a hollow tube that allows for fluid drainage from or injection into an area.

Clean intermittent catheterization

The placement of a catheter into the bladder to drain urine and the removal after the urine is drained at defined intervals throughout the day to allow for bladder emptying. It may also be performed to maintain patency after treatment of a bladder neck contracture or urethral stricture.

The advantages of clean intermittent catheterization are that it allows you to know when you are able to void on your own, it minimizes bladder and urethral irritation, and it has less risk of infections and bladder stones over the long term.

give you a sufficient trial because of the increased risk of urinary incontinence.

Urinary Incontinence

Urinary incontinence is uncommon in men undergoing interstitial seed therapy. In men who have not had a prior TURP, incontinence occurs in less than 1%. In men who have had a prior TURP, the risk of incontinence is 25% and is up to 40% if more than one TURP has been performed.

Rectal Ulceration/Bleeding

Rectal irritation does not occur as commonly as urinary symptoms and tends to improve quicker than urinary symptoms. Less than 5% of patients will have a rectal ulcer or rectal bleeding, which occurs as a result of irritation of the rectal lining. It may be associated with pain, rectal spasms, and the feeling that one needs to have a bowel movement. This condition can be treated with several topical medications, including Anusol, hydrocortisone, Proctofoam hydrocortisone, mesalamine (Rowasa) suppositories, Metamucil, and a low-roughage diet.

PSA "Bounce" or "Blip"

This occurs when the PSA increases on two consecutive blood draws and then decreases and remains low without rising again. The cause of this phenomenon is not known. It occurs in about one third of men treated with interstitial seeds and typically occurs around 9 to 24 months after the treatment. It may or may not be accompanied by symptoms of prostate inflammation; if such symptoms are present, then treatment for prostatitis may decrease the symptoms and the PSA level. Some advocate that after brachytherapy, to avoid unnecessary active interventions after surgery that the PSA levels be monitored for at least 3 years and to provide reassurance to patients that a PSA rise during this time is common and may not indicate treatment failure.

Urethral Stricture

This narrowing of the urethra is related to the development of scar tissue; it is uncommon after interstitial seeds, occurring in 5–12% of men, and tends to develop later. It may present with a change in the force of stream or the need to strain to void. A stricture is identified by cystoscopy in the doctor's office. Treatment of the stricture depends on the location and the extent of the stricture; it may require a simple office dilation or an incision under anesthesia.

Erectile Dysfunction

This condition may occur in as many as 40% to 60% of men who undergo interstitial seed therapy. Unlike radical prostatectomy, the erectile dysfunction tends to occur a year or more after the procedure and not right away. There is an increased risk of post–seed therapy erectile dysfunction in older men and in those receiving hormone therapy. Erectile dysfunction after interstitial seed therapy responds well to a variety of treatment options (see Question 91).

59. Who is a candidate for interstitial seed therapy?

Similar to radical prostatectomy, the goal of interstitial therapy is to cure one of prostate cancer. With this in mind, the candidate should have a life expectancy of more than 7 to 10 years so that he will benefit from a cure and no underlying illness that would contraindicate performing the procedure. Men with significant obstructive voiding symptoms and/or prostate volumes greater than 60 mL are at increased risk for voiding troubles and urinary retention after the procedure. Men who have undergone a prior TURP are at increased risk for urinary incontinence after brachytherapy. Men with clinically localized prostate cancer of low to intermediate risk are candidates for interstitial seed therapy. Men with high-risk prostate cancer (PSA > 20 ng/mL, Gleason score > 8, or stage T3a prostate cancer) should not be treated with interstitial seed therapy alone. The use of combination therapy—androgen deprivation therapy (ADT) plus interstitial seed therapy—is recommended for men with favorable intermediate-risk as well as high-risk prostate cancer.

60. What happens the day of the procedure and what can I expect?

Your physician will give you instructions regarding your diet for the day or two before the procedure. You may be asked to have a clear liquid diet the day before the procedure and to use an enema to clean out stool from the rectum the evening before the procedure. As with any surgical procedure, you will be instructed not to eat or drink after midnight the evening before surgery. You may take your medications with a sip of water. The brachytherapy procedure is performed under anesthesia, either spinal or general. After adequate anesthesia has been obtained, you are placed in a dorsal lithotomy position. You are lying on your back, with your legs bent, elevated, and separated to allow access to the perineum and rectum. A Foley catheter is placed through the urethra into the bladder, and a small amount of contrast material (X-ray dye) is placed into the balloon of the catheter so that the balloon can be visualized under **fluoroscopy**, which involves the use of a fluoroscope, a radiologic device used for examining deep structures by means of X-rays. The catheter allows the doctor to identify where the **bladder outlet** is.

Fluoroscopy

Use of a fluoroscope, a radiologic device that is used for examining deep structures by means of X-rays.

Bladder outlet

The first part of the natural channel through which urine passes when it leaves the bladder.

The bladder outlet is the first part of the natural channel through which urine passes when it leaves the bladder. The prostate sits right below the outlet.

A repeat TRUS is performed to measure the volume of the prostate again and to determine the number of needles and corresponding radioactive seeds, the isotope and the isotope strength necessary for the procedure. The seeds may be placed into the prostate through a variety of techniques including fluoroscopic guidance, ultrasound guidance, or via the use of an MRI. At the end of the procedure the catheter is removed, and a cystoscopy (a look into the bladder with a telescope-like device) may be performed to make sure that no seeds are in the bladder or urethra. If seeds are found in the bladder or urethra, they are removed.

A catheter is often placed after the cystoscopy is performed, and the patient is discharged to home with the catheter in place for 24 hours. After the procedure is completed and the patient has recovered, a CT scan is obtained and CT-based dosimetry is calculated to assess the seed placement and the dose of radiation delivered throughout the prostate.

Several terms are used to describe the dose of radiation. The D100 is the dose received by the entire prostate, the V100 is the percent of the volume of the prostate that received 100% of the prescribed dose, and the V150 is the percent of the volume of the prostate that received 150% of the prescribed dose. An acceptable seed implantation should maintain a V100 of at least 80%. Although the D100 is often below the prescribed dose as a result of the sharp decrease in the radiation dose at the edge of the implant, ideally the total dose should be about 90% of the D100 (D90).

You may also notice some blood in the urine after the procedure; this is related to urethral irritation and usually resolves within 24 hours.

Ejaculation

The release of semen through the penis during orgasm. After radical prostatectomy and often after a TURP, no fluid is released during orgasm.

Semen

The whitish fluid that is released during ejaculation.

Testis

One of two male reproductive organs that are located within the scrotum and produce testosterone and sperm.

After the procedure is performed, you may notice some swelling, black and blue coloring, or slight bleeding from the perineum (the area under the scrotum and in front of the anus). This is related to the needle placement and usually resolves over the next few days. The area may also be tender to touch; applying ice packs intermittently to the area for the first 24 hours after the procedure helps decrease the swelling, and sitz baths, nonsteroidal anti-inflammatory drugs, and Tylenol help reduce the discomfort. Good personal hygiene minimizes infection.

You may also notice some blood in the urine after the procedure; this is related to urethral irritation and usually resolves within 24 hours. There may also be some blood in the fluid released during **ejaculation** (the release of **semen** through the penis during orgasm), the ejaculate; in fact, the ejaculate may look brown, black, or even red after the procedure. This may seem alarming, but it is not cause for concern. The ejaculate is composed of fluid from the **testis**, the prostate, and the seminal vesicles. Thus, bleeding in the prostate or seminal vesicles that results from needle penetration may cause blood in the ejaculate, which resolves with time.

61. When can I return to work after interstitial seed therapy?

Because the procedure is minimally invasive and requires no incisions, you can typically return to work and full activity within 3 to 4 days after the procedure.

62. If I have had brachytherapy, am I a radiation risk to others?

No. Although the seeds are radioactive, you are not, and thus you are not a radiation risk to others. The seeds emit radiation, but the vast majority of the radiation is absorbed by the prostate. Intimate contact will not pass on the radiation. However, some recommend that for the first two months after seed placement, you should limit contact with small children and pregnant women.

63. Why is my radiation oncologist or urologist recommending interstitial seed therapy plus EBRT?

Interstitial seed therapy is limited in its ability to reach tissue outside of the prostate, especially the back of the prostate. The addition of EBRT may help in patients who are judged to be at high risk for disease penetrating through or outside the prostate capsule. Use of interstitial seeds alone is appropriate for patients with tumors in clinical stage T1c to T2a, a Gleason score < 6, and a PSA < 10. Patients with a Gleason score of 7 or greater, a PSA > 10, tumors in clinical stage T2b or minimal T3a, and at least four of six biopsies positive for cancer or perineural invasion on the biopsy appear to be the best served by the combination of interstitial seeds and EBRT.

Current AUA/ASTRO guidelines recommend a combination of ADT and EBRT for men with intermediate- and high-risk prostate cancer.

64. Where can I find out who performs brachytherapy in my area, and how do I choose the appropriate individual to perform the brachytherapy?

You could call your local hospital and ask whether they have a listing of urologists/radiation oncologists that perform interstitial seed therapy in your area. When you discuss brachytherapy with the urologist or radiation oncologist, you may wish to ask several questions, including:

1. How long has the physician been performing brachytherapy, and how many procedures has he or she performed?
2. What is the individual's success and failure rate?
3. What is his or her complication rate?
4. What does the physician feel is your likelihood of success or failure and your likelihood of complications given your PSA level, Gleason grade, and overall health?

65. How am I monitored after interstitial seed placement?

Unlike with radical prostatectomy, the prostate remains in your body, and thus the PSA does not decrease to an undetectable level. In addition, it may take at least 2 years for the PSA to reach its lowest level (**PSA nadir**). The PSA is typically checked 1 month after seed placement and then every 3 to 6 months for 2 years thereafter if the level remains stable. After 2 years, the PSA is checked yearly. Failure of seed therapy is defined as a nadir of < 0.5 ng/mL to 1.0 ng/mL or three consecutive rises in the PSA level more than 3 months apart for each value. A rise in PSA may occur in as many as one third of the patients between the first and second year after the implantation. This is called a "benign PSA bump," and it appears to be related to late tissue reactions to the radiation; it does not mean that the seeds have failed or that you are at increased risk of failure. In this situation, the PSA does not continue to rise, and this is how one differentiates a PSA bump from a failure.

PSA nadir

The lowest value that the PSA reaches during a particular treatment.

66. What is the success rate of brachytherapy?

The results of prostate brachytherapy are comparable to those of radical prostatectomy for 5 to 7 years after treatment. The long-term data (i.e., the data for longer than 10 years after treatment) are limited. Reported studies demonstrate success rates of 64% to 85% at 10 years, with success being defined by either a PSA < 0.5 ng/mL or the absence of three consecutive rises in PSA in patients who received brachytherapy EBRT. Pretreatment nomograms have been developed to help physicians and patients estimate the probability of successful treatment 5 years after brachytherapy including CAPRA score and ProCaRS. A 12-year study of patients treated with brachytherapy alone or with external-beam radiation therapy (EBRT) demonstrated that 66% of the patients who underwent brachytherapy alone and 79% who underwent brachytherapy plus EBRT were free of PSA or clinical recurrence.

67. What are external-beam and conformal external-beam radiation therapy? What are the side effects of EBRT? What is CyberKnife radiation therapy?

External-beam radiation therapy (EBRT) is the use of radiation therapy to kill or inactivate cancer cells. The total radiation dose is given in separate individual treatments, known as "fractionation." Cancer cells are most sensitive to radiation at different phases in their growth. By giving the radiation on a daily basis, the radiation oncologist hopes to catch the cancer cells in the sensitive phases of growth and also to prevent the cells from having time to recover from the radiation damage. Conformal EBRT uses CT images and sophisticated computer software to help better visualize the radiation targets and the normal tissues; with 3D images, the radiation oncologist can identify critical structures, such as the bladder, the rectum, and the hip bones. This allows the radiation oncologist to deliver more radiation (72–82 Gy as opposed to 66–72 Gy with standard EBRT) to the prostate tissue but decrease the amount of normal tissue that is irradiated. The advantage of conformal EBRT over EBRT is that conformal EBRT causes less rectal and urinary irritation. The construction of an immobilization device (cradle) and the placement of small, permanent tattoos ensure that you are properly positioned for the radiation treatment each day. Through the assistance of computers, the radiation oncologist can define an acceptable dose distribution to the prostate and surrounding tissues, and the computer determines the appropriate beam configuration to create this desired distribution.

Intensity modulated therapy (IMRT)

An advanced form of 3D conformal radiation.

Intensity-modulated therapy (IMRT) is the newest way of administering EBRT. IMRT uses hundreds of tiny radiation beam-shaping devices to deliver a single dose of radiation. The collimators can be stationary or move during treatment. This kind of dose modulation allows different areas of a tumor or nearby tissue to receive different doses of radiation. Studies have demonstrated that high-dose (81 Gy) IMRT is well tolerated and associated with excellent long-term tumor control in patients with localized prostate cancer.

The side effects of EBRT or conformal EBRT can be either acute (occurring within 90 days after EBRT) or late (occurring > 90 days after EBRT). The severity of the side effects varies with the total and the daily radiation dose, the type of treatment, the site of treatment, and the individual's tolerance. The most commonly noted side effects include changes in bowel habits, bowel bleeding, skin irritation, edema, fatigue, and urinary symptoms, including dysuria, frequency, hesitancy, and nocturia. Less commonly, swelling of the legs, scrotum, or penis may occur. Late side effects include persistence of bowel dysfunction, persistence of urinary symptoms, urinary bleeding, urethral stricture, and erectile dysfunction.

Bowel Changes

A change in bowel habits is one of the more common side effects of EBRT. Patients may develop diarrhea, abdominal cramping, the feeling of needing to have a bowel movement, rectal pain, and bleeding. Usually, if these side effects are going to occur, they do so in the second or third week of treatment.

If diarrhea is severe enough to warrant treatment, you can use loperamide (Imodium), paregoric, attapulgite (Kaopectate), or diphenoxylate HCl with atropine sulfate (Lomotil). Changes in dietary habits, such as eating a low-residue diet and avoiding certain foods (milk, raw vegetables, squash, gas-producing vegetables, dried fruit, fiber cereals, seeds, popcorn, nuts, chunky peanut butter, corn, and dried beans) are helpful. Drinking plenty of fluids helps prevent dehydration.

Rectal pain can be treated with warm sitz baths, hydrocortisone-containing creams (Proctofoam HC, Cortifoam), or anti-inflammatory suppositories (Tucks, Rowasa).

Late bowel effects include persistent changes in bowel function, rectal **fistula** (a communication between the rectum and other site, e.g., the prostate or the skin), or

Fistula

An abnormal passage or communication, usually between 2 internal organs, or leading from an internal organ to the surface of the body.

perforation (a hole in the rectum), and bleeding. Rectal fistula and perforation are rare and often require surgical treatment.

Skin Irritation

The tolerance of the skin to radiation depends on the dose of radiation used and the location of the skin affected. Certain areas are more sensitive than others; the perineum and the fold under the buttocks are very sensitive and may become red, flake, or drain fluid. To prevent further irritation, avoid applying soaps, deodorants, perfumes, powders, cosmetics, or lotions to the irritated skin. After you wash the area, gently blot it dry. Cotton underwear and loose-fitting clothes can help prevent further irritation. If the irritated skin is dry, topical therapies can be applied, such as petroleum jelly (Vaseline), lanolin, zinc oxide, Desitin, Aquaphor, Proctofoam, and corn starch.

Edema

Edema of the legs, scrotum, and penis may rarely occur, but when it does, it is more common in those who have undergone prior pelvic lymph node dissection. Lower-extremity edema can be treated with supportive stockings, TED hose, and elevation of feet when sitting and lying down. Penile and scrotal edema is often difficult to treat.

Urinary Symptoms

The genitourinary symptoms of dysuria, frequency, hesitancy, and nocturia are related to changes that occur in the bladder and urethra that result from radiation exposure. The bladder may not hold much urine because of the irritation and scarring, and irritation of the bladder lining may make it more prone to bleeding. Bladder inflammation usually occurs about 3 to 5 weeks into the radiation treatments and gradually subsides about 2 to

8 weeks after the completion of radiation treatments. Urinary anesthetics (phenazopyridine HCL [Pyridium]) and bladder relaxants (flavoxate HCl [Urispas], hyoscyamine sulfate [Cystospaz], oxybutynin [Ditropan], and tolterodine [Detrol]), or other anticholinergics may be helpful in decreasing the urinary frequency.

CyberKnife

The CyberKnife Robotic Radiosurgery System is the most widely used form of prostate stereotactic body radiation therapy (SBRT). SBRT is like external beam therapy, but the radiation is given over fewer visits and at higher doses. It is indicated for men with low-risk prostate cancer. In the clinical trials, low-risk prostate cancer was defined as PSA < 10 ng/mL, Gleason score of 3 + 3 (or low-volume Gleason 3 + 4), and clinical stage T1c, T2a, or T2b. In a study of 304 patients followed for a median of 5 years post treatment, 97% of patients with low-risk prostate cancer and 90.7% of patients with intermediate-risk prostate cancer remained cancer-free throughout the follow-up. Side effects of CyberKnife typically resolve one month after treatment and include dysuria, urgency, frequency, nocturia, and tenesmus (a continual or recurrent feeling of the need to have a bowel movement). Medicare coverage of CyberKnife appears to vary by geographic location and insurance coverage appears to be variable.

68. Who is a candidate for EBRT, conformal EBRT, and IMRT?

Similar to other curative treatments, the ideal patient has a life expectancy of 7 to 10 years. In higher-risk patients, the increased radiation dose used with conformal EBRT causes a significantly better decrease in PSA progression than the dose used in conventional EBRT. EBRT is also an option for men with lower-risk prostate cancer who have a high probability of progression on active surveillance. EBRT is recognized as a treatment option for men with intermediate- and high-risk prostate cancer, and the AUA/ASTRO guidelines recommend the addition of ADT for such individuals. There does not appear to be a PSA **progression-free survival** benefit with conformal EBRT when compared with conventional EBRT in patients who have low-risk prostate cancer. Men who have a PSA level > 10 ng/mL or with a tumor that is clinical stage T3 are the most likely to benefit from the higher radiation doses that can be achieved with conformal EBRT and may benefit from combination therapy, such as hormone therapy plus EBRT. The amount of radiation and the field of radiation differ for each individual and depend on the clinical stage and the Gleason grade. Contraindications to EBRT include a history of inflammatory bowel disease, such as Crohn's disease and ulcerative colitis, or a history of prior pelvic radiotherapy.

Progression-free survival

The length of time during and after treatment during which the disease being treated (cancer) doesn't progress (get worse).

69. What does the treatment entail?

Conformal EBRT requires that you undergo a treatment planning session (simulation) that includes a CT scan. Thereafter, you are seen five days a week (Monday through Friday) for a short period of time to receive a treatment. The treatments last for about 6 to 7 weeks, depending on the total dose selected by your radiation oncologist. The dose received and the use of neoadjuvant or adjuvant therapy may vary with your risk factors. Hormonal therapy is often recommended for men with a Gleason score of 7 or higher or a PSA of 10 ng/mL or higher in conjunction with standard dose EBRT (about 70 cGy) or dose escalation to 78–79 cGY using 3D conformal radiation technique. IMRT delivers doses as high as 81 Gy. In low-risk patients, dose escalation appears to be beneficial. In intermediate-risk patients, either a short course (about 6 months) of hormone therapy and standard dose EBRT or dose escalation is recommended. The regimen varies according to your clinical stage and whether the radiation therapy is being given as a firstline therapy or as a secondary therapy, such as for an increasing PSA after radical prostatectomy.

Use of Radiation Therapy After Radical Prostatectomy

The ASTRO and AUA published a joint guideline on radiation therapy after prostatectomy for patients with and without evidence of prostate cancer. Highlights from this publication include: (1) Patients with adverse pathologic findings including seminal vesical invasion, positive surgical margins, and extraprostatic extension (i.e., prostate cancer cells into the fat around the prostate) should be informed that adjuvant radiation therapy (EBRT), compared to radical prostatectomy alone, reduces the risk of biochemical (PSA) recurrence, local recurrence, and clinical progression of cancer; (2) salvage radiation therapy should be offered to patients with PSA or local recurrence after radical prostatectomy in whom there is no evidence of distant metastatic disease; and (3) the effectiveness of radiation therapy for PSA recurrence is greatest when given at lower levels of PSA.

70. What is the success rate of EBRT or conformal EBRT?

The success rate varies with the initial PSA level. In one study, 89% to 92% of men treated with conformal EBRT whose pretreatment PSA was < 10 ng/mL showed no increase in PSA level at 5 years. Those with a pretreatment PSA of 10 to 19.9 ng/mL had an 82% to 86% chance of no increase in PSA level at 5 years, compared with a 26% to 63% chance of no increase in PSA at 5 years in men with a pretreatment PSA of > 20 ng/mL.

Men with T1 and T2 tumors have survival rates that are comparable to that with radical prostatectomy. In such individuals, the clinical tumor-free survival is 96% at 5 years and 86% at 10 years.

71. What is cryotherapy/cryosurgery? What are the complications of cryotherapy?

Cryotherapy is a technique used for prostate cancer treatment that involves controlled freezing of the prostate gland.

Cryotherapy is a technique used for prostate cancer treatment that involves controlled freezing of the prostate gland. First-line cryotherapy treatment is an option, when treatment is appropriate, for men with a negative metastatic evaluation. The size of the prostate gland affects the ability to obtain uniform freezing of the prostate and individuals with large prostates may benefit from decreasing the size of the prostate by the use of pretreatment hormone therapy. This procedure is performed under anesthesia. TRUS evaluation (similar to that used with your prostate biopsy) is used throughout the procedure to visualize the prostate and to monitor the position of the freezing probes, which are placed through the perineal skin (the area below the scrotum and in front of the anus) into the prostate (**Figure 14**, page 121). During the freezing, the TRUS demonstrates an "ice ball" in the prostate. The freezing process kills both hormone-sensitive and hormone-insensitive cancer cells. Proper positioning of the probe may allow one to kill cancer cells even at the edge of the prostate, the prostate capsule.

Cryotherapy is performed under TRUS guidance. Cryoneedles/probes are placed through the skin into the prostate. TRUS allows for visualization of the edge of the frozen tissue as a hyperechoic rim with acoustic shadowing, in addition, thermocouples record when lethal temperatures are reached in the prostate as well as evaluating temperatures in sensitive adjacent structures such as the rectum and sphincter. Urethral warming can help decrease the risk of urethral sloughing.

Argon-based cryosurgery allows for rapid temperature drops in the prostate and the user of thinner cryoneedles/probes. The use of helium gas, which warms when it expands, provides a warming capacity that was not available with earlier forms of cryotherapy. Critical to cryotherapy is rapid freezing of the prostate tissue. In addition, double-freeze thaw cycle is recommended as it is believed that those cancer cells not killed by the first freeze cycle are sufficiently stressed so that a second cycle is lethal. The freeze cycle should be at least 220°C and historically a target of 240°C is recommended.

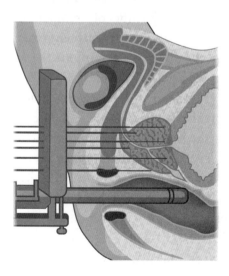

Figure 14
Placement of needles for cryoablation of the prostate.
Courtesy of Endocare.

72. Who is a candidate for cryotherapy?

Although more commonly used as a **salvage** therapy (a procedure intended to "rescue" a patient after a failed prior therapy) for men who fail to respond to EBRT or interstitial seeds, cryotherapy can be used as a first-line therapy in individuals who have clinically organ-confined disease of any grade with a negative metastatic evaluation. The AUA/ASTRO guidelines note that low-risk prostate cancer patients considering whole prostate cryotherapy need to be aware that side effects of this treatment are considerable and the survival benefit has not been compared to active surveillance. The guidelines note that cryotherapy is an option for select intermediate-risk localized prostate cancer and do not recommend cryotherapy for high-risk prostate cancer. (To review the best practice policy on cryosurgery and/or the recent AUA/ASTRO guidelines on clinically localized prostate cancer, see www.auanet.org.) High-risk patients may, however, require multimodal therapy. The size of the prostate gland is a factor in patient selection and outcome. The larger the prostate the more difficult it is to achieve a uniformly cold temperature throughout the gland. Thus, those men with large prostates may benefit from the addition of hormone therapy (GnRH agonist or antagonist) to decrease the size of the prostate prior to cryotherapy. A relative contradiction to preforming cryotherapy is a large TURP defect. Cryotherapy achieves the best results when the starting PSA is < 10 ng/mL. Cryotherapy is a minimally invasive option when treatment is appropriate for men who either don't want or who aren't good candidates for radical prostatectomy because of comorbidities such as obesity or a history of pelvic surgery. It may also be a reasonable option for men with a narrow pelvis or those who cannot tolerate EBRT and those with previous nonprostatic pelvic irradiation, inflammatory bowel disease, or rectal disorders. For patients desiring minimally invasive therapy for intermediate-risk prostate cancer, Gleason 7 or 8 with PSA > 10 ng/mL and < 20 ng/mL or clinical stage T2b, cryotherapy is also an option.

More recently, investigators have looked at "focal cryotherapy" as opposed to "whole gland cryotherapy" as a potential of treating focal, localized prostate cancer while decreasing the impact of treatment on sexual function and bowel function. An analysis of the national CryOn-Line Database (COLD) registry involving 5,853 patients, of whom 1,160 underwent focal cryotherapy, demonstrated that the biochemical recurrence free-rate (ASTRO definition) at 36 months was 75.7%. Urinary continence, as defined by the lack of pad usage, was 98.4%, and 58.1% of patients noted maintenance of spontaneous erections.

The role of focal cryotherapy remains investigative and the results of long-term studies are needed to assess the feasibility and efficacy of this therapy. Critical to its success are reliable methods to identify focal areas of prostate cancer to treat and post-treatment follow-up regimens, given the limitations of PSA after treatment.

73. What is the success rate of cryotherapy?

In the case of cryosurgery, there is no universally accepted biochemical measure of failure. Because the urethra is preserved, there is always the possibility of PSA producing tissue being preserved. In this situation, the PSA will not decrease to an undetectable level. However, it is felt that the lower the nadir PSA, the greater the probability of a negative biopsy and stable post-treatment PSA over time.

In patients who have not responded locally to EBRT, approximately 40% who then undergo salvage cryotherapy have an undetectable PSA level after cryotherapy, and 78% have negative prostate biopsy results. It appears that a drop in the PSA to 0.5 ng/mL after cryotherapy is associated with a good prognosis. In men with post-cryotherapy PSA levels > 0.5 ng/mL, there is a higher likelihood that the PSA will increase or that the prostate biopsy result will be positive. When cryotherapy is used as the initial primary therapy, a PSA lowest value of ~0.5 ng/mL is associated with a better prognosis.

In studies with long-term data ranging from 5–10 years post cryotherapy, the 5-year biochemical disease for survival rates for low-, intermediate-, and high-risk cases range from 65–92%, 69–89%, and 48–89%, respectively.

A multicenter registry (the COLD registry) of primary cryotherapy (no prior surgery or radiation-based procedures) reported pool 5-year biochemical (PSA) disease-free progression outcomes, noting that:

- 85% of low-risk patients are disease-free at 5 years
- 73.4% of intermediate-risk patients were disease-free at 5 years
- 75% of high-risk patients were disease-free at 5 years

The above results were obtained using the old ASTRO biochemical disease-free definition. Using the "Phoenix" definition of nadir PSA plus 2 ng/mL (Roach et al., *Int J Radiat Oncol Biol Phys.* 2006;65(4):965–974), the following results were achieved:

- 91% biochemical disease-free rate in low-risk patients
- 78% biochemical disease-free rate in intermediate-risk patients
- 62% biochemical disease-free rate in high-risk patients

What Are the Side Effects/Complications of Cryotherapy?

The complications of cryotherapy appear to be related to the effects of the freezing on surrounding tissues and can be minimized by careful TRUS monitoring and urethral warming during the procedure. Most individuals undergoing cryotherapy are undergoing the treatment as a salvage procedure after failed radiation therapy. The radiation effects on the surrounding tissues leave the tissue with limited reserve for healing and repair, thus increasing the risk of complications. Common side effects of cryotherapy include perineal pain, transient urinary retention, penile and/or scrotal swelling, and hematuria. Urinary retention occurs in roughly 3% of individuals. Anti-inflammatories seem to help, but individuals may require a catheter or suprapubic tube for a few weeks post-treatment. Penile and/or scrotal swelling is common in the first or second post-procedure weeks and usually resolves within 2 months of cryotherapy. Penile paresthesia may occur and usually resolves within 2 to 4 months post-procedure. Long-term complications of cryotherapy include: fistula formation, incontinence, erectile dysfunction, and urethral sloughing. With cryotherapy directed at the entire prostate gland, the external urinary sphincter is inevitably affected by the freeze, although it is somewhat protected by the urethral warming catheter. Thus, there is a risk of urinary incontinence with cryotherapy and when present it is usually limited to mild stress incontinence. The risk of permanent incontinence (i.e., need to wear a pad) is reported to range from < 1% to 8%. However, in individuals undergoing salvage cryotherapy after radiation failure, the incidence of urinary incontinence may be as high as 43%. Similarly, with total prostate gland cryotherapy, the ice ball extends beyond the capsule of the prostate and in most cases encompasses the neurovascular bundles and can cause erectile dysfunction. The incidence of erectile dysfunction after cryotherapy in the literature ranges from 49% to 93% at 1-year post-cryotherapy. However, potency rates of 51.3% have been reported at 4 years post-treatment with the use of penile rehabilitation post-cryotherapy. The risk of fistula formation, a connection between the prostate and the rectum, occurs in 0% to 0.5% of individuals undergoing cryotherapy for prostate cancer and is highest in those men undergoing salvage cryotherapy after failed radiation therapy (EBRT). Urethral sloughing occurs less frequently with use of the urethral warming catheter. Urethral sloughing may cause dysuria and urinary retention. Symptomatic patients may require transurethral resection of the necrotic tissue. The incidence of urethral sloughing after cryotherapy with the use of the urethral warming catheter ranges from 0% to 15%. Symptomatic patients may require transurethral resection of the necrotic tissue.

74. What options are available if primary cryotherapy does not help me?

If the failure occurs locally within the prostate and there is no sign of cancer outside of the prostate, then a radical prostatectomy could technically be performed. The risks of incontinence and impotence associated with radical prostatectomy after cryotherapy are significant. Hormone therapy is also an option in patients with a rising PSA after primary cryotherapy.

75. Are there different types of hormone therapy/androgen deprivation therapy (ADT)? Do I need to have my testicles removed?

Hormone therapy is a form of prostate cancer treatment designed to decrease the production of the male hormones (androgens such as testosterone and dihydrotestosterone) and their action on the prostate cancer cells. **Hormones** are substances that are responsible for secondary sex characteristics, such as hair growth and voice changes in males. **Androgens** are necessary for the development and function of the male sexual organs and male sexual characteristics (e.g., hair, voice change). The most common androgen is **testosterone**. Androgens are primarily produced by the testicles, under control of various parts of the brain. A small amount of androgen is produced by the adrenal glands, which are small glands located above the kidneys and which produce many important chemicals. Prostate cancer cells may be hormone sensitive, hormone insensitive, or castrate-resistant. Cancer cells that are hormone sensitive require androgens for growth. Thus, elimination of the androgens would prevent the growth of such cells and cause them to shrink. Normal prostate cells are also hormone sensitive and also shrink in response to hormone therapy. Prostate cancer cells that are castrate-resistant have adapted to be able to grow despite a very low testosterone level as a result of hormone therapy, but remain sensitive to testosterone.

Hormone therapy is not a "curative" therapy, because it does not kill the prostate cancer cells; rather, it is "palliative" in that its goal is to slow down the progression, or growth, of the prostate cancer. Hormone therapy for patients with metastatic disease may work effectively for

Hormones

Substances (estrogens and androgens) responsible for secondary sex characteristics (hair growth and voice change in men).

Androgens

Hormones that are necessary for the development and function of the male sexual organs and male sexual characteristics (i.e., hair, voice change).

Testosterone

The male hormone or androgen that is produced primarily by the testes and is needed for sexual function and fertility.

Hormone therapy is not a "curative" therapy, because it does not eliminate the prostate cancer cells; rather, it is "palliative" in that its goal is to slow down the progression, or growth, of the prostate cancer.

Neoadjuvant therapy

The use of a treatment, such as chemotherapy, hormone therapy, and radiation therapy, before surgery.

several years; however, over time, the castrate-resistant cells will emerge, and the cancer will grow.

Hormone therapy may be used as a primary, secondary, or neoadjuvant therapy. Hormone therapy is often used as a primary therapy in older men who are not candidates for surgery or radiation therapy and who are not interested in watchful waiting (see Question 83). It is also used in men who have metastatic disease at the time that their prostate cancer is detected. Men who experience a continuous rise in their PSA after radical prostatectomy, radiation therapy, or cryotherapy are given hormone therapy to slow down the growth of the recurrent prostate cancer. Lastly, hormone therapy may be given for a period of time before radical prostatectomy or radiation therapy to shrink the prostate gland and make the procedure easier to perform (**neoadjuvant therapy**). Neoadjuvant therapy has a significant impact on the pathology, such that it is very difficult for the pathologist to grade the cancer cells after 3 months of hormone therapy.

In men with recurrent prostate cancer after EBRT or radical prostatectomy or in those who do not have organ-confined prostate cancer at the time of diagnosis, the time at which hormone therapy should be started is not clear. For this reason, one must weigh the potential benefits and side effects of hormone therapy. Hormone therapy may delay disease progression, but its effect on survival does not appear to be significant. In one study in men with prostate cancer, delaying hormone therapy for 1 year was associated with an 18% increase risk of death due to prostate cancer; although this was a large study, it is still only one study, and more information is needed.

Many different forms of hormone therapy exist, and they may be subdivided into two groups: surgical and medical therapies. The surgical approach is a bilateral **orchiectomy** (removal of both testicles), whereby the main source of androgen production, the testicles, are removed.

Bilateral orchiectomy is performed in men with prostate cancer to remove most of the male hormone (testosterone) production. Typically, this procedure can be performed as a minor surgical procedure under local anesthesia. Depending on the urologist's preference, it can be performed through a single incision in the middle of the scrotum or through two incisions, one on each side of the scrotum. The blood vessels that supply the testis and the sperm duct (the vas deferens) are tied off, and the testes are removed. Some urologists perform a subcapsular orchiectomy, whereby the testicular tissue is removed from within the outer coat (the capsule), and the capsule remains in the scrotum, leaving some fullness to the scrotum. To minimize swelling and bleeding in the scrotum, the scrotum is often wrapped to compress it or a scrotal supporter is used to elevate it. The incision is closed with dissolvable sutures so that the stitches will not need to be removed.

The advantages of bilateral orchiectomy are that it causes a quick drop in the testosterone level (the testosterone level drops to its lowest level by 3 to 12 hours after the procedure [average is 8.6 hours]), it is a one-time procedure, and it is more cost effective than the shots, which often require several office visits per year and are more expensive. The disadvantages of orchiectomy are those of any surgical procedure and include bleeding, infection, permanence, and scrotal changes. In men who have undergone bilateral orchiectomy and are bothered by an "empty" scrotum, bilateral testicular prostheses may be placed that are the same size as the adult testes. Most men who undergo bilateral orchiectomy lose their

Orchiectomy
Removal of the testicle(s).

TREATMENT OF PROSTATE CANCER

Bilateral orchiectomy is performed in men with prostate cancer to remove most of the male hormone (testosterone) production.

libido and have erectile dysfunction after the testosterone level is lowered. Other long-term side effects of bilateral orchiectomy, related to testosterone depletion, include hot flushes, osteoporosis, fatigue, loss of muscle mass, anemia, and weight gain.

Medical therapy is designed to stop the production of androgens by the testicles and the effects of androgens on the prostate cancer cells. There are three types of medical therapies: **gonadotropin-releasing hormone (GnRH) agonists**, **antiandrogens**, and **GnRH antagonists**. These prevent the action of testosterone on the prostate cancer and on normal prostate cells (antiandrogen), or prevent the production of testosterone from the testes (GnRH). GnRH agonists and antagonists are very effective in lowering the testosterone level.

Gonadotropin-Releasing Hormone Agonists

The brain controls testosterone production by the testicles. GnRH agonists are chemicals produced in the brain that in turn stimulate the production of another chemical produced by the brain, GnRH. GnRH tells the testicles to produce testosterone. Initially, when a man takes a GnRH agonist, there is an increased production of LH and of testosterone. This superstimulation in turn tells the brain to stop producing GnRH and, subsequently, the testicles stop producing testosterone. It takes about 5 to 8 days for the GnRH agonists to drop the testosterone levels significantly. The increase in testosterone that may occur initially with GnRH agonists may affect patients with bone metastases, and there may be a worsening of their bone pain called the **flare reaction**. Such men with metastatic disease will be given another medication, an antiandrogen, for 2 weeks or so before starting the GnRH agonist to block the effects of the testosterone and to prevent the flare phenomenon.

Gonadotropin-releasing hormone (GnRH) agonists

A class of drugs that prevent testosterone production by the testes.

Antiandrogen

A medication that eliminates or reduces the presence or activity of androgens.

GnRH antagonist

A form of hormone therapy that works at the level of the brain to directly suppress the production of testosterone without initially raising the testosterone level.

Flare reaction

A temporary increase in tumor growth and symptoms that is caused by the initial use of GnRH agonists. It is prevented by the use of an antiandrogen 1 week before GnRH agonist therapy begins.

GnRH agonists are given as shots either monthly, every 3 months, every 4 months, every 6 months, or yearly. There are five forms of GnRH agonists: leuprolide acetate for intramuscular injection (Lupron Depot®), triptorelin pamoate suspension for intramuscular injection (Trelstar Depot and Trelstar LA), leuprolide acetate for subcutaneous injection (Eligard), histrelin acetate for subcutaneous implant (Vantas), and goserelin acetate implant (Zoladex). They work in essentially the same way but differ in how they are given (**Table 8**, pages 133–134). The advantage of this form of therapy is that it does not require removal of the testicles, it is not permanent, and the newer longer-acting-formulations require less frequent office visits. However, it is more expensive than bilateral orchiectomy over the long term. If you miss a shot, your testosterone level increases, and the prostate cancer cells may grow; thus, it is important to get the shots on a regularly scheduled basis. If you are traveling, you can plan ahead and contact doctors in areas where you will be to arrange for the shots.

Gonadotropin-Releasing Hormone Antagonists

Degarelix (Firmagon) is a GnRH antagonist that was demonstrated in clinical trials to rapidly decrease serum testosterone (within 3 days) and is not associated with the initial surge of testosterone and risk of flare that is seen with GnRH agonist. The starting dose is 240 mg given as two subcutaneous injections of 120 mg and then maintenance doses of 80 mg as one subcutaneous injection every 28 days. Phase III studies have demonstrated that degarelix is at least as effective as leuprolide in sustaining castrate levels or lower of testosterone and had a statistically significant faster decrease in testosterone levels.

GnRH agonists/antagonists have side effects that may affect your quality of life over the short and long term. Some of the side effects related to these medications, such as hot flushes, erectile dysfunction (see Question 91), anemia, and osteoporosis, can be treated. Erectile dysfunction occurs in about 80% of men taking GnRH agonists/antagonists and is associated with decreased libido (sexual desire). The widely prescribed drug sildenafil (Viagra) as well as the other oral therapies for erectile dysfunction, vardenafil (Levitra) and tadalafil (Cialis), are effective in most of these men if they had normal erectile function before starting hormone therapy. Unfortunately, there is no medication to restore libido.

Osteoporosis is loss of bone density, and it leads to weakened bones that break more easily.

A recent Gallup survey of American men revealed that most men believe that osteoporosis is a "women's disease." **Osteoporosis** is loss of bone density, and it leads to weakened bones that break more easily. Yet this disease can affect men, particularly men taking hormone therapy for prostate cancer. If you have risk factors for decreased bone mineral density, your doctor may want to check your bone density before starting **androgen deprivation therapy** (**ADT**). It is anticipated that there will be approximately 2,000 osteoporosis-induced fractures in men with advanced prostate cancer.

Risk factors include:

- *Family history*: patients with a family history of decreased bone density have a 50% or higher increased risk of developing osteoporosis.
- *Increased age*: most men and women lose about 0.5% bone mass every year after age 50 years.
- *Lifestyle related*: decreased calcium and vitamin D, smoking, excessive alcohol consumption, caffeine intake, or lack of exercise.
- *Diseases associated with bone loss*: chronic obstructive pulmonary disease (COPD), malabsorption syndrome, hyperparathyroidism, **hypogonadism**, renal insufficiency, and vitamin D deficiency.

Osteoporosis

The reduction in the amount of bone mass, leading to fractures after minimal trauma.

Androgen deprivation therapy (ADT)

A treatment based on the reduction of androgen hormones, which stimulate prostate cancer cells to grow.

Hypogonadism

In males, a condition in which the testes do not produce enough testosterone.

Table 8 Commonly Used Antiandrogens and GnRH Analogues

Agent	Dose	Route of Administration	Action	Side Effects
Lupron Depot ® (leuprolide acetate for depot injection)	7.5 mg/mo 22.5 mg/3 mos 30 mg/4 mos 45 mg/6 mos	IM	GnRH agonist	Impotence, decreased libido, osteoporosis, anemia, hot flushes, weight gain, fatigue, flare phenomenon. Long-term use may prolong the QT interval.
Eligard (leuprolide acetate for injectable suspension)	7.5 mg/mo 22.5 mg/3 mos 30 mg/4 mos 45 mg/6 mos	SQ	GnRH agonist	Same as Lupron.
Trelstar Depot/LA (triptorelin pamoate injectable suspension)	3.75 mg/mo 11.25 mg/3 mos 22.5 mg/6 mos	IM	GnRH agonist	Same as Lupron.
Vantas (histrelin acetate implant)	50 mg/yr	SQ	GnRH agonist	Same as Lupron.
Zoladex (goserelin)	3.6 mg/mo 10.8 mg/3 mos	SQ	GnRH agonist	Same as Lupron.

(continues)

Table 8 Commonly Used Antiandrogens and GnRH Analogues (continued)

Agent	Dose	Route of Administration	Action	Side Effects
Firmagon (degarelix)	240 mg given as two injections of 120 mg each as initial dose, followed 28 days later by maintenance dose of 80 mg every 28 days	SQ	GnRH antagonist	Injection site reactions, hot flush, impotence, weight gain, fatigue, increase in transaminases, HTN, chills. Long-term use may prolong the QT interval.
Eulexin (flutamide)	750 mg/day	PO	Antiandrogen	Breast tenderness and enlargement, hot flushes, diarrhea, anemia, abnormal liver function.
Nilandron (nilutamide)	300 mg/day for 30 days, then 150 mg daily	PO	Antiandrogen	Same as with Eulexin. Also, reversible lung disease, alcohol intolerance, decreased night vision.
Casodex (bicalutamide)	50 mg/day	PO	Antiandrogen	Same as with Eulexin.

Abbreviations: mos, months; PO, orally; SQ, subcutaneously; comb rx, combination treatment; IM, intramuscularly.

How can you tell if osteoporosis is occurring? The best way to check the bone mineral density is the dual-energy X-ray absorptiometry (DEXA) scan, the same study used to evaluate for osteoporosis in women. It is **noninvasive** (i.e., it does not require an incision or the insertion of an instrument or substance into the body), precise, and a quick test that involves minimal radiation exposure. The test measures the bone mineral density, which is compared with values obtained from normal, young, adult control subjects. The controls have been well established for women but need to be better defined for men. In addition, there appears to be an ethnic variability in bone density, with African-American males usually having higher peak bone mass and a lower risk of osteoporotic fractures than Caucasian males. Normally, the bone mineral density is at its highest by age 25, and after age 35 both men and women lose 0.3% to 0.5% of their bone mass per year as part of the normal aging process. Men have a higher peak bone mass than women.

Several factors contribute to loss of bone mineral density, but decreased sex hormone production has the most significant impact on bone mineral density. Low testosterone levels affect bone mineral density in men almost the same as low estrogen levels in women. The use of ADT, whether it be via orchiectomy or GnRH agonist/antagonist with or without antiandrogens, causes decreased bone mineral density. There is an average loss of 4% per year for the first 2 years on hormone therapy and 2% per year after year 4, which is similar to the loss in women after removal of the ovaries or natural menopause. This loss of bone mineral density in men taking hormone therapy occurs for at least 10 years and probably accounts for the increased incidence of fractures: 5% to 13.5% of men taking hormone therapy have fractures compared to 1% in men with prostate cancer who are not receiving hormone therapy.

Noninvasive

Not requiring any incision or the insertion of an instrument or substance into the body.

TREATMENT OF PROSTATE CANCER

Lifestyle modifications that may help decrease the risks of bone complications in men on hormonal therapy include: smoking cessation, decreased alcohol intake, performing weight bearing and arm exercises, and taking supplements of 1,200 mg of calcium and 400 to 800 international units of vitamin D daily. Calcium-rich diets include dairy products, salmon, spinach, and tofu.

When should men on hormone therapy be evaluated for osteoporosis? There are no good guidelines to help determine how frequently DEXA scans should be obtained in men with prostate cancer who are taking hormone therapy. It may be helpful to obtain a baseline DEXA scan before starting hormone therapy and then obtain periodic DEXA scans thereafter. What can be done to prevent or treat osteoporosis? Several studies have shown that an increase in bone mineral density loss occurs in men who have had an orchiectomy compared to men who are receiving GnRH agonist/antagonist. The reason for this is not clear, but this result suggests that other chemicals are produced by the testes that may be important in maintaining bone density. Further studies may help identify these chemicals. Certain factors can put one at increased risk for osteoporosis, including sedentary lifestyle, decreased sun exposure, glucocorticoid therapy, excess caffeine intake, decreased dietary calcium and vitamin D intake or exposure, increased salt intake, aluminum-containing antacid consumption, alcohol abuse, smoking, family history of decreased bone mineral density, and diseases associated with bone loss including COPD, malabsorption syndrome, hyperparathyroidism, hypogonadism, renal insufficiency, and vitamin D deficiency.

Diethylstilbestrol (DES)

A form of the female hormone estrogen.

Changes in lifestyle can help prevent osteoporosis. Low-dose estrogen therapy, **diethylstilbestrol (DES)**, 1 mg per day, has been shown to be helpful in stabilizing the loss of bone mineral density, but it has the risk of blood clots.

Another group of medications that are more commonly used in women with osteoporosis are the biphosphonates, which prevent bone breakdown. Three different biphosphonates, alendronate (Fosamax), neridronate (Nerexia), and zoledronate (Zometa), have been used to prevent osteoporosis in androgen-deficient men with prostate cancer. Zoledronate is FDA approved and has been shown to increase bone density in men on hormonal therapy. In a small study, pamidronate (Avedia) used in combination with leuprolide was shown to preserve bone density in men with prostate cancer on leuprolide hormone therapy.

Denosumab (Prolia, Xgeva) 60 mg has been shown to have a significant effect on bone mineral density compared to placebo in men with nonmetastatic prostate cancer and decreases the risks of new vertebral fractures. Denosumab is not a biphosphonate; it is a monoclonal antibody that is injected under the skin every 6 months. Denosumab is FDA approved for treatment to increase bone mass in men at high risk for fracture receiving ADT for nonmetastatic prostate cancer. It can cause severe lowering of the calcium levels. It may also cause fatigue, decreased phosphate levels, and nausea. Calcium and vitamin D supplementation may be needed to prevent **hypocalcemia** (low calcium level in the blood).

Hypocalcemia
Low calcium level in the bloodstream.

Selective estrogen modulators (SERMs) including raloxifene and toremifene have been shown to improve bone mineral density in men on ADT, but remain investigational. They are approved for the prevention of osteoporosis in postmenopausal women.

Another way of potentially decreasing the risk of osteoporosis is the use of intermittent hormone therapy. However, whether intermittent ADT may decrease bone mineral density remains controversial. With this form of therapy, you are on and off the hormones for set periods of time. The idea of intermittent hormone therapy is that the prostate cancer cells that survive while you are on hormone therapy (hormone insensitive) become hormone sensitive again when they are exposed to androgens. Possible advantages of intermittent androgen suppression include preservation of androgen sensitivity of the tumor, improved quality of life because of recovery of libido and potency and improved sense of well-being, and decrease in treatment cost. In the non-metastatic setting, intermittent ADT has been shown to be just as effective as continuous ADT.

The long-term effects of intermittent hormone therapy are not well known. The duration that one receives the hormone therapy, the time to restart hormone therapy, how to tell whether the disease is progressing, and who is the ideal patient for intermittent hormone therapy are not well defined. One potential way to give intermittent androgen suppression therapy (androgen blockade) is shown in **Figure 15** (page 139).

Staying Healthy on ADT

Use of hormone therapy (androgen deprivation therapy) may affect lean muscle mass, fat mass, bone health, cholesterol levels, and insulin resistance. Currently, there are no set guidelines for definitive management of such adverse effects. However, there are several "healthy living" changes that you can institute to help prevent or decrease the severity of such effects.

1. Exercise is important. Regular exercise three times a week can decrease fatigue and improve muscle fitness and quality of life.

2. Eat healthy and follow your cholesterol levels. Because high cholesterol is a common problem in adults overall, it may be helpful to have your

cholesterol level checked before you start hormone therapy, within 1 year after starting the hormone therapy, and periodically thereafter. If your cholesterol levels are high and dietary changes are not effective, talk to your primary care doctor about medications to treat high cholesterol.

3. Resistance to insulin is a risk factor for diabetes and heart disease. Use of hormone therapy may increase insulin resistance. Some physicians recommend having a fasting blood glucose and/or hemoglobin A1C (a test checking long-term blood sugar levels) prior to starting hormone therapy, within 1 year after starting hormone therapy, and periodically thereafter. If your hemoglobin A1C is between 6–6.5% or you

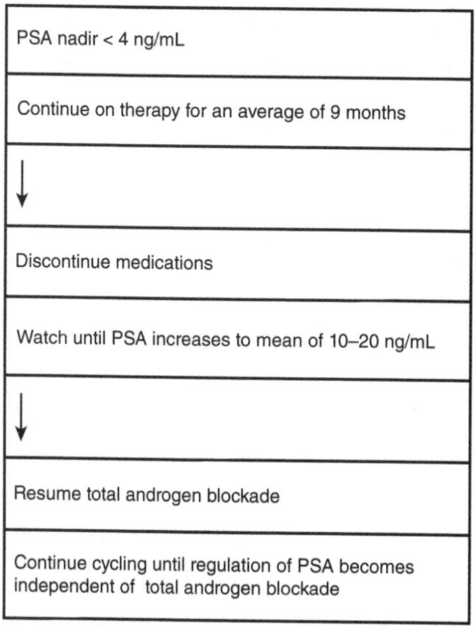

PSA nadir < 4 ng/mL
Continue on therapy for an average of 9 months
↓
Discontinue medications
Watch until PSA increases to mean of 10–20 ng/mL
↓
Resume total androgen blockade
Continue cycling until regulation of PSA becomes independent of total androgen blockade

Figure 15 Intermittent androgen blockage.

Data from Miyamoto H, Messing EM, Chang C. Androgen deprivation therapy for prostate cancer: current status and future prospects. *Prostate*. 2004;61(4): 332-53; Hussain M, Tangen C, Berry D et al. Intermittent versus continuous androgen deprivation for prostate cancer. *NEJM*. 2013; 268(14):1314–1325.

have an impaired fasting glucose (fasting glucose 100–125 mg/dL) you are at increased risk for developing diabetes and should pursue 5-10% weight loss and participate in moderate physical exercise for at least 2.5 hours or more per week (*J Natl Compr Canc Netw.* 2010;8(2): 211–223).

✔ Eat healthy
- Avoid foods high in saturated fats

✔ Exercise regularly
- At least 150 minutes per week

✔ Watch your weight

✔ Talk with your doctor about calcium and vitamin D supplements to help maintain healthy bones

✔ Ask your doctor if low-dose aspirin is appropriate for you

✔ Have your blood sugar and hemoglobin A1c followed

✔ Consider a test to measure your bone density and therapies to maintain bone health

---

GnRH agonist/antagonists often are used alone as primary, secondary, or neoadjuvant therapy. Over time, the PSA level may increase. When the PSA increases, your doctor may check your serum testosterone level to make sure that the GnRH agonist/antagonist is dropping the testosterone level to almost undetectable levels. In some cases with the use of the GnRH agonist/antagonist on an every 3- to 4-month basis, the testosterone suppression may not be adequate, and switching to a more frequent dosing interval, such as an every 28-day formulation, may be more effective. When a man is receiving hormone therapy, the testosterone level should be ≤ 20 ng/dL. When the PSA increases despite GnRH agonist/antagonists, the GnRH agonist/antagonists are continued, and another medication, an antiandrogen, is added. This combined therapy is called total androgen blockade and is often effective in treating the prostate cancer for 3 to 6 months.

Antiandrogens

Antiandrogens are **androgen receptor blockers**; they prevent the attachment of the androgens, both those produced by the testicles and those produced by the adrenal glands, to the prostate cancer cells, thus preventing them from acting on these cells. Because these chemicals do not actually affect testosterone production, the testosterone level remains normal or may be slightly elevated if they are used alone. Thus, these medications do not affect libido or erectile function when they are used alone. However, antiandrogens are not commonly used alone; rather, they are used in combination with GnRH agonist/antagonist. One antiandrogen, bicalutamide (Casodex), has been shown to be effective in the treatment of prostate cancer by itself, but it is not approved by the FDA for monotherapy. There are three commonly used antiandrogens: bicalutamide (Casodex), flutamide (Eulexin), and nilutamide (Nilandron). As with all medications, these medications have side effects, which are listed in **Table 9** (page 142) (see Question 76). When antiandrogens are used in combination with GnRH agonist/antagonist, this is called **total (maximal) androgen blockade**. Total androgen blockade is used for individuals whose PSA increases significantly while they are taking GnRH agonist/antagonists.

A new androgen receptor blocker, enzalutamide (Xtandi), has been approved by the FDA. Unlike the older forms of androgen receptor blockers, it works in multiple ways, but currently is only indicated in patients with metastatic castrate-resistant prostate cancer (see Questions 77 and 81).

Androgen receptor blocker

A chemical that binds to the androgen receptor preventing the binding of androgens (testosterone and dihydrotestosterone).

Total (maximal) androgen blockade

The total blockage of all male hormones (those produced by the testicles and the adrenal glands) using surgery and/or medications.

Antiandrogens are androgen receptor blockers; they prevent the attachment of the androgens, both those produced by the testicles and those produced by the adrenal glands, to the prostate cancer cells, thus preventing them from acting on these cells.

TREATMENT OF PROSTATE CANCER

Table 9 Drugs Commonly Used in Treating Hot Flushes

Drug	Dosage	Possible Side Effects
Megestrol acetate (Megace)	20 mg BID	Chills, appetite stimulation, weight gain
Clonidine (Catapres)	0.1 mg patch each week	Hypotension, skin reaction
Medroxyprogesterone Acetate (Provera or Depo-Provera)	400 mg IM or 25 mg PO BID	Cardiovascular side effects
Venlafaxine	12.5 mg PO BID	Depression, nausea, loss of appetite
Cyproterone acetate	50 mg PO TID	Rarely, tumor may grow; cardiovascular side effects
Diethylstilbestrol (DES)	1 mg PO QD	Cardiovascular side effects, difficult to obtain, blood clots

Abbreviations: BID, twice a day; TID, three times a day; IM, intramuscularly; PO, orally; QD, every day.

Hot flushes occur in men receiving hormone therapy for the treatment of high-stage prostate cancer and in patients receiving neoadjuvant hormone therapy.

Hot flushes

The sudden feeling of being warm, may be associated with sweating and flushing of the skin, which occurs with hormone therapy.

76. Why do hot flushes occur with hormone therapy, and can they be treated?

Hot flushes occur in men receiving hormone therapy for the treatment of high-stage prostate cancer and in patients receiving neoadjuvant hormone therapy (hormone therapy administered before definitive treatment, e.g., radical prostatectomy or interstitial seeds to shrink the prostate cancer).

In a study of men receiving neoadjuvant therapy before radical prostatectomy, **hot flushes** (a sudden feeling of being warm, which may be associated with sweating and flushing of the skin) occurred in 80% of the patients. In about 10%, the hot flushes continued for at least 3 months after they stopped the hormone therapy. Men who received hormone therapy for > 4 months were more likely to have hot flushes that persisted. Approximately three quarters (75%) of the men being treated with hormone therapy for prostate cancer report bothersome hot flushes that begin 1 to 12 months after starting hormone therapy and often persist for years. The hot flushes may vary in intensity and can last from a few seconds to an hour.

The cause of hot flushes and sweating (vasomotor symptoms) associated with hormone therapy (shots or orchiectomy) is not well known. The symptoms are similar to those that women experience while going through menopause, yet they are not typically experienced by men, whose testosterone level slowly declines with aging. The symptoms appear to be related to the sudden large decrease in the testosterone level and the effects that testosterone has on blood vessels. There are no identifiable factors that put one individual at higher risk for hot flushes than another.

There are many ways to treat hot flushes associated with hormone therapy, and different men respond to different treatments (Table 9, page 142). Some options include clonidine (a blood pressure medication), the hormone megestrol acetate (Megace), estrogen patches, low-dose estrogen (DES), and medroxyprogesterone acetate (Provera, DepoProvera). Oral estrogen has been effective in getting rid of the hot flushes; however, estrogen use carries the risk of heart problems, strokes, and blood clots. Low-dose Megace has been used effectively to treat hot flushes and works in about 85% of people. However, it has been associated in rare cases with an increase in PSA that decreased with stopping the Megace and thus must be used cautiously. Another chemical, cyproterone acetate, has been used to treat hot flushes, but it is associated with cardiac side effects, is expensive, and is not approved for this use by the FDA. The hormone, Provera, given orally or intramuscularly, has been effective in treating hot flushes, but it also may have some cardiovascular side effects. The anti-depressant venlafaxine (Effexor), medroxyprogesterone acetate (Provera; a progestin), and cyproterone acetate all were shown to decrease the number and intensity of hot flushes in a trial of over 300 men receiving hormonal therapy for advanced prostate cancer. In women, clonidine patches have been helpful in decreasing the incidence and severity of hot flushes with natural or surgically induced (hysterectomy and removal of the ovaries) menopause, but they do not appear to be as effective in men. Eating a serving of soy daily in addition to 800 IU of vitamin E in one study was shown to decrease the number and the severity of hot flushes to 50%. You should not take this amount of vitamin E without consulting your medical doctor first. Lastly, the anticonvulsant drug gabapentin and antidepressants like venlaxafine have been shown to be useful in treating hot flushes. Limiting caffeine intake and avoiding strenuous exercise and very warm temperatures are also helpful in controlling hot flushes.

Castrate-resistant prostate cancer (CRPC)

Prostate cancer that is resistant to hormone therapy and resultant low (< 20 ng/dL) testosterone level.

Metastatic castrate-resistant prostate cancer (mCRPC)

Prostate cancer that continues to progress despite ADT and castrate levels of testosterone and has spread to sites outside of the prostate, commonly the lymph nodes and bones.

77. What are castrate-resistant prostate cancer (CRPC) and metastatic castrate-resistant prostate cancer (mCRPC) and how are they treated?

Castrate-resistant prostate cancer (CRPC) is a term used to apply to prostate cancer that is growing despite ADT, as demonstrated by a rising PSA, with or without evidence of metastatic disease. If there is metastatic disease (i.e., spread to the lymph nodes and/or bones), then it is called **metastatic castrate-resistant prostate cancer (mCRPC)**.

CRPC is thought to develop by changes in the prostate cancer cells that allow them to grow despite low levels of testosterone. The androgen receptor, the area on the prostate cancer cell where androgens (testosterone and dihydrotestosterone) bind, is very important in the growth of prostate cancer cells. As prostate cancer cells become castrate-resistant there are several changes which occur with the androgen receptor and overall:

- There is an increase in the number of androgen receptors, making it easier to bind to more testosterone.
- There may be a change in the androgen receptor that allows other chemicals to bind to it or that allows it to function even better (magnifies) when testosterone binds to it.
- There may be changes in the androgen receptor or its function.
- The prostate cancer cells may develop the ability to produce their own testosterone.
- The older forms of androgen receptor blockers actually may act to stimulate the androgen receptor, instead of block it, over the course of time.
- The prostate cancer cells may develop new ways to grow that don't involve the androgen receptor.

In clinical terms, CRPC is the progression of prostate cancer in patients with castrate levels of testosterone (< 20 to 50 ng/mL). To put this in perspective, mid-normal range testosterone levels in young, healthy men are 400–700 ng/mL, while normal testosterone levels in older men are slightly lower. This progression might be the result of an increase in PSA levels (PSA progression) reflecting growth of the cancer cells or metastases (the spread of cancer cells to areas in the body outside of the prostate gland, commonly the lymph nodes and bones; see Figure 4, page 35).

The Prostate Cancer Clinical Trials Working Group defines asymptomatic, non-metastatic CRPC as an increase in PSA level both 2 ng/mL above and 25% higher than the PSA nadir (the lowest level of PSA that the patient had during treatment). This must be confirmed by a second PSA at least 3 weeks later, in the absence of metastatic disease.

The European Association of Urology (EAU) definition of CRPC states that the following must occur:

- The patient must have a testosterone level ≤ 50 ng/mL plus either.
- There must be 3 consecutive increases in the PSA levels, 1 week apart, resulting in two 50% increases over the nadir. Or,
- Radiological progression—appearance of 2 or more bone lesions on bone scan or enlargement of a soft tissue lesion.

Performance status

An attempt to quantify cancer patients' general well-being and activities of daily life.

The AUA recommends observation with continuation of the GnRH agonist/antagonist in men with asymptomatic CRPC. When mCRPC develops a variety of options are available for treatment (**Figure 16**, page 147, and **Table 10**, page 148–152). The indications for use of the different therapies may vary depending on the severity of symptoms, **performance status**, and prior therapies. Because the prostate cancer cells remain sensitive to hormones in most individuals, the ADT (LHRH agonist/antagonist) is *continued* while other therapies are added. There have been several new therapies developed, many of which may be used when one fails a prior therapy. Each of these therapies have been demonstrated to improve quality of life and prolong survival by several months. Unfortunately, to date none of these therapies cure prostate cancer, but research continues in hopes of developing such a therapy. A new therapy, apalutamide (Erleada) an androgen receptor blocker, has been recently approved in 2018 for treatment of nonmetastic castrate resistant prostate cancer. It is to be used in conjuction with a GnRH analog or bilateral orchiectomy. Further information can be obtained from https://www.accessdata .fda.gov/drugsatfda_docs/label/2018/210951s000lbl.pdf.

78. What is immunotherapy/vaccine therapy for prostate cancer?

Vaccine therapy involves the injection of a chemical, an antigen, into an individual. The antigen stimulates the individual's body to produce cells that fight off the antigen, and in doing so, kill the cancer cells. Several different vaccines are being investigated. Sipuleucel-T (Provenge) is the only one currently that is FDA approved; it is used for mCRPC in men who are asymptomatic or minimally symptomatic.

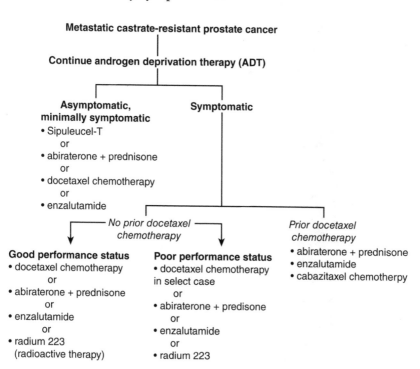

Figure 16 Treatment options for metastatic castrate-resistant prostate cancer.

Taxane(s)

A chemotherapy drug derived from the yew tree that prevents cell growth by inhibiting special cell structures, called microtubules, which are involved in cell division.

Prednisone

A synthetic (man-made) drug that is similar to corticosterone.

Alopecia

Partial or complete loss of hair from parts of the body where it normally grows (baldness).

Sensory neuropathy

Damage to the nerves of the peripheral nervous system that can cause abnormal sensations, like tingling or a prickling feeling.

Stomatitis

Inflammation of the lining of the mouth.

Table 10 Treatment Options for Metastatic Castrate-Resistant Prostate Cancer

Therapy and Approved Indication	Dosing	Effect on Overall Survival	Other Effects	Side Effects
First-line chemotherapy: taxane (docetaxel) *Indication:* CRPC and mCRPC	Intravenous over 60 minutes every 3 weeks plus **prednisone.**	19.2 months compared to 16.3 with an older form of chemotherapy.	Reduction in pain, rates of PSA level response higher, and better quality of life than older form of chemotherapy.	*Contraindication:* prior hypersensitivity to taxane or polysorbate, neutrophil count < 1,500 cells/mm^3. *Warning/Caution:* may affect heart conduction and rarely require pacemaker placement, use with caution with concomitant use of medications that affect the CYP2C8 and CYP3A4 enzymes, hypersensitivity reactions may occur resulting in shortness of breath, low blood pressure, angioedema and urticaria, may cause liver toxicity, fluid retention, and toxic death. *Side effects:* neutropenia, fatigue, **alopecia**, nausea/vomiting, diarrhea, nail changes, **sensory neuropathy,** changes in taste, **stomatitis,** abnormal liver function tests.

Therapy and Approved Indication	Dosing	Effect on Overall Survival	Other Effects	Side Effects
Second-line chemotherapy: taxane (cabazitaxel) *Indication:* mCRPC refractory to first-line taxane	Intravenous over 60 minutes every 3 weeks plus prednisone.	15.1 months compared to 12.7 months for older form of chemotherapy.	Significantly better progression free survival, decrease in tumor, and decrease in PSA level.	*Contraindication:* prior hypersensitivity to taxane or polysorbate, neutrophil count < 1,500 cells/mm³. *Warning/Caution:* may affect heart conduction and rarely require pacemaker placement, use with caution with concomitant use of medications that affect the CYP2C8 and CYP3A4 enzymes, hypersensitivity reactions may occur resulting in shortness of breath, low blood pressure, angioedema and urticaria, may cause liver toxicity, fluid retention and toxic death. Caution regarding use in patients with elevated bilirubin. *Side effects:* neutropenia, fatigue, alopecia, nausea/vomiting, diarrhea, nail changes, sensory neuropathy, changes in taste, stomatitis, abnormal liver function tests, **thrombocytopenia.**

(continues)

Thrombocytopenia
A decrease in the platelet count of the blood.

Table 10 Treatment Options for Metastatic Castrate-Resistant Prostate Cancer (continued)

Therapy and Approved Indication	Dosing	Effect on Overall Survival	Other Effects	Side Effects
Immunotherapy/ Vaccine therapy: sipuleucel-T (Provenge) *Indication*: asymptomatic or minimally symptomatic mCRPC	Each cycle involves removal of blood, harvesting and activation of specialized immune cells, and reinfusion. A complete course is 3 cycles, each cycle separated by 2 weeks.	3.7 to 4.5 months for immunotherapy compared to placebo.	Time to progression of the cancer was 0.2 weeks to 2.6 weeks longer with immunotherapy than placebo. There was no significant difference in reduction of PSA by at least 50% between immunotherapy and placebo.	Most common side effects include chills, fever, fatigue, nausea, joint ache, and headache, which usually occur within first few days of treatment.
CYP17 inhibitor: abiraterone (Zytiga) (inhibitor of androgen production by testes, adrenal glands, and prostate cancer cells) *Indication*: mCRPC	Four 250 mg tablets orally once a day, on an empty stomach, plus prednisone 5 mg orally twice a day.	15.8 months compared to 11.2 months for placebo in patients who had received prior first-line chemotherapy; in patients with mCRPC who did not receive prior	Significant radiographic progression-free survival was noted with CYP17 inhibitor compared to placebo. The PSA response rate was 38% with CYP17 inhibitor compared to 1.0% with placebo and progression-free survival was 5.6 months with CYP17 versus 3.6 months with placebo. Significant delayed chemotherapy and significant delayed opioid use.	*Warning/Caution*: Use with caution in patients with heart disease; monitor for signs and symptoms of adrenal insufficiency; may need to increase doses of prednisone during stressful situations; may cause hypertension and hypokalemia; monitor liver function for signs of liver toxicity; should not be used in patients with severe liver impairment; may be affected by concomitant use of other

Therapy and Approved Indication	Dosing	Effect on Overall Survival	Other Effects	Side Effects
CYP17 inhibitor: abiraterone (Zytiga) (*continued*)		chemotherapy, 35.3 months compared to 30.1 months with placebo.		medications that affect CYP3A4 and CYP2D6 enzymes. *Side effects:* fatigue, joint swelling or discomfort, edema, hot flushes, diarrhea, vomiting, cough, shortness of breath, urinary tract infection, bruising, hypertension, **hypokalemia**, high blood sugar, high cholesterol, abnormal liver function tests, hypophosphatemia, muscle discomfort.
Androgen Receptor Inhibitor: enazlutamide (Xtandi) *Indication:* mCRPC	Four 40 mg (160 mg) capsules once a day, with or without food.	18.4 months compared to 13.6 months with placebo in patients with mCRPC after first-line chemotherapy.	Greater percentage of patients with PSA decrease of 50% or more, better reduction in soft tissue metastases, better quality of life with androgen receptor inhibitor compared to placebo in patients with mCRPC after first-line chemotherapy. Time to PSA progression 8.3 months versus 3.0 months with placebo.	*Warning/Caution:* may be affected by concomitant use of medications that affect CYP2C8, CYP3A4, CYP2C9, and CYP2C19 enzymes. Has not been studied in patients with history of seizures. *Side effects:* **asthenia**, fatigue, back pain, diarrhea, arthralgia, hot flush, edema of lower extremities, muscle

(continues)

Hypokalemia

Low potassium level in the bloodstream.

Asthenia

Abnormal physical weakness or lack of energy.

Table 10 Treatment Options for Metastatic Castrate-Resistant Prostate Cancer (continued)

Therapy and Approved Indication	Dosing	Effect on Overall Survival	Other Effects	Side Effects
Androgen Receptor Inhibitor: enazlutamide (Xtandi) *Indication:* mCRPC *(continued)*			Time to first skeletal related adverse event 16.7 months compared to 13.3 months with placebo in patients with mCRPC with prior trial first-line chemotherapy.	pain, headache, **upper and lower respiratory tract infections,** muscle weakness, dizziness, insomnia, spinal cord compression, blood in the urine, **paresthesia,** anxiety, high blood pressure, seizure.
Radionuclide therapy: Radium 223 (Xofigo) *Indications:* Symptomatic mCRPC with bone metastases, without visceral metastases	50KBq per kg/body weight given at 4-week intervals for 6 injections.	14.9 months for radionuclide compared to 11.3 months for placebo.	Time to first symptomatic skeletal event significantly longer with radionuclide therapy, 15.6 months compared to 9.8 months for placebo. Reduces pain.	*Warning/Caution:* therapy can cause significant bone marrow suppression—measure blood counts before starting therapy and before each treatment. *Side effects:* nausea, diarrhea, vomiting, peripheral edema, anemia, low white blood cell count, low platelet count.

For complete information on a particular drug, please refer to the prescribing information provided by the drug manufacturer.

Provenge is developed from one's own blood. A sample of blood is drawn and sent to a specialized laboratory where it is processed to extract certain cells called antigen-presenting cells (APCs). The cells are then "activated" when cultured with a protein, prostate acid phosphatase-GMCSF, which consists of **prostatic acid phosphatase (PAP)** an antigen expressed in prostate cancer tissue linked to **granulocyte macrophage colony-stimulating factor (GMCSF)** which "activates" the immune cells. The mixture is then injected back into your blood over the course of an hour. This process is repeated three times over approximately 3 weeks.

Studies have demonstrated that individuals with mCRPC treated with Provenge immunotherapy lived 4 months longer than patients with mCRPC who received a placebo in a trial.

79. Are there therapies that block testosterone production from the adrenal glands as well as the testicles?

Abiraterone (Zytiga) is a **CYP17 inhibitor** (Table 10, pages 148–152). CYP17 is an enzyme found in the adrenal glands and the testes which is necessary for the production of testosterone and other chemicals in the body. Zytiga is given along with a steroid, prednisone, for the treatment of mCRPC and it works by blocking the production of testosterone in both the adrenal glands and the testes. The recommended dose is 1,000 mg (four 250-mg tabs) taken orally once a day in combination with prednisone 5 mg twice a day, on an empty stomach (no food 2 hours before or 1 hour after the dose). The most common side effects of Zytiga are: joint swelling or discomfort, low potassium (hypokalemia), muscle aches, hot

Upper respiratory tract infection

An acute infection involving nose, sinuses, and throat.

Paresthesia

Abnormal sensation, typically tingling or prickling, that could be due to nerve damage.

Prostatic acid phosphatase (PAP)

An antigen produced by prostate cancer cells.

Granulocyte macrophage colony-stimulating factor (GMCSF)

A protein secreted by several cells that stimulates the growth and development of various cells.

CYP17

An enzyme in the adrenal gland and testes that is needed for testosterone production and other chemicals.

CYP17 inhibitor

An inhibitor of the CYP17 enzyme in the testes and adrenal glands, which is needed for testosterone production.

TREATMENT OF PROSTATE CANCER

flush, diarrhea, urinary tract infection, cough, hypertension (high blood pressure), arrhythmia (irregular heart beat) frequency, nocturia, dyspepsia, and upper respiratory tract infection (URI). Some of the side effects are related to the build up of mineralocorticoids, which cause fluid retention. Patients taking abiraterone are at risk for adrenal insufficiency (lack of production of other important chemicals by the adrenal glands) and thus prednisone must be taken along with the abiraterone.

In a clinical trial compared to placebo, Zytiga prolonged life by a median of about 4 months.

80. Is chemotherapy used for prostate cancer? What are the side effects?

Chemotherapy refers to the use of powerful drugs to either kill cancer cells or interfere with their growth. Several different drugs have been shown to improve symptoms and cells, though no drug has been shown to cure prostate cancer. Ongoing clinical trials continue to look for new chemotherapy drugs and combinations of drugs in hopes of finding more effective and less toxic options. Several drugs have been tried in the treatment of mCRPC including estramustine, vinblastine, and mitoxantrone as well as a group of drugs called the taxanes. Currently, the taxanes—docetaxel and more recently cabazitaxel—are the most commonly used chemotherapy drugs, both as first-line and second-line chemotherapy for mCRPC (see Table 10, pages 148–152).

Taxanes are drugs that are derived from the yew tree. They affect the growth of prostate cancer cells by affecting their microtubules, preventing the cells from dividing. They have been shown to improve survival in men with mCRPC. Docetaxel is the first-line chemotherapy drug. It has been shown to improve survival and quality of life, as well as provide better pain control in men with mCRPC than another chemotherapy drug, mitoxantrone. Another taxane, cabazitaxel (Jetvana), has been approved by the FDA for treatment of mCRPC in men who have failed docetaxel. In a Phase III trial of 755 patients, cabazitaxel was used as a second-line chemotherapy and increased survival by 28% compared to mitoxantrone chemotherapy. Men who received cabazitaxel had a median survival of 15.1 months compared to 12.7 months for those receiving mitoxantrone.

Side effects of the taxanes include: fluid retention; dry skin; thickened, discolored nails; weight gain; and decreased blood cell production. Docetaxel is given intravenously, often in combination with a steroid, prednisone, which helps minimize some of the side effects.

81. The androgen receptor is very important in the growth of prostate cancer; are there any new therapies that affect the androgen receptor?

Androgen receptor blockers (antiandrogens) have been used for some time in men with an increasing PSA on GnRH agonist/antagonist therapy as part of combined or maximal androgen therapy. This combined therapy has been shown to be effective in slowing down the growth of prostate cancer and increases overall survival by about 3% to 5% at 5 years compared to monotherapy with a GnRH agonist/antagonist. However, the prostate cancer cells eventually develop the ability to grow despite combination therapy. In the development of CRPC, there appear to be several changes that occur with the androgen receptor. First, there is an increase in the number of androgen receptors, improving the ability of the cancer cells to bind what little testosterone is present. Second, the androgen receptor appears to develop the ability to bind testosterone more tightly, increasing the chance that the androgen receptor–testosterone complex will be moved into the center of the cell (the nucleus) and stimulate the production of chemicals essential for the growth of the prostate cancer cells. In addition, changes in the structure of the androgen receptor may lead to the older forms of androgen receptor blockers (antiandrogens) acting as stimulants. It is thought that this combination of increased number of androgen receptors, tighter binding of androgen (testosterone/dihydrotestosterone) to the androgen receptor, and enhanced movement of the androgen–androgen receptor complex into the nucleus of the prostate cancer cell results in a 10,000-fold decrease in the amount of testosterone needed for prostate cancer cell growth.

Enzalutamide (Xtandi) is a new androgen receptor blocker recently approved by the FDA (Table 10, pages 148–152). It differs from the older forms of androgen receptor blockers (antiandrogens) as it binds more tightly to the androgen receptor, preventing the binding of testosterone/dihydrotestosterone. It also prevents the movement of this complex into the nucleus of the cell and prevents the complex from interacting with the DNA in the nucleus, thus preventing production of the chemicals needed for cell growth. Thus, this new androgen receptor blocker prevents the growth of prostate cancer cells by three mechanisms instead of one. In addition, it does not act as a stimulant over the course of time, unlike the older forms of androgen receptor blockers. Currently, enzalutamide is approved as a first-line therapy for the treatment of mCRPC. It has been shown to prolong survival by about 4.8 months compared to placebo in patients for whom chemotherapy has been ineffective.

The dose of enzalutamide is 160 mg (four 40-mg capsules) once a day, with or without food. Side effects of enzalutamide include: asthenia, fatigue, back pain, diarrhea, arthralgias, hot flushes, muscle pain, headaches, muscle weakness, dizziness, rarely seizure, and other side effects related to prostate cancer disease progression.

82. What is gene therapy for prostate cancer? Are there other therapies under investigation?

Prostate cells become malignant because of gene changes in the cells. The goal of gene therapy is to place genes into the cancer cells that would cause the cancer cells to return to their normal state or would cause the cancer cells to die. Various centers throughout the United States are running clinical trials using gene therapy: The Johns Hopkins University School of Medicine, UCLA Medical Center, Duke University Medical Center, University of Michigan School of Medicine, Dana Farber Cancer Institute, Baylor College of Medicine, Mt. Sinai School of Medicine, Vanderbilt University Medical Center, and MD Anderson Cancer Center.

83. What are watchful waiting/ observation and active surveillance?

Watchful waiting/observation is the decision not to treat the prostate cancer at the time of diagnosis and is not aimed at curing one of prostate cancer, but rather to institute palliative treatment for local or metastatic disease progression if it occurs. It is based on the premise that some patients will not benefit from definitive treatment for the primary prostate cancer. Rather than treat the cancer, the physician monitors the PSA value at various intervals to assess whether it is increasing and at what rate (the PSA velocity). Ideally, the patient and the physician identify a point at which therapy would be instituted (for example, a PSA value of a certain number or the presence of bone pain), and the patient is monitored without therapy until he changes his mind or that point is reached. Watchful waiting differs from active surveillance in that with active surveillance one is followed more closely and the intent is to intervene while the prostate cancer may still be treated definitively.

Watchful waiting is ideally suited for patients with potentially life-threatening medical conditions and older patients with low Gleason scores.

Watchful waiting is ideally suited for patients with potentially life-threatening medical conditions and older patients with low Gleason scores. In these individuals, it is less likely that prostate cancer will be the cause of their death. Younger (< 72 years) men, healthy men, and those with a higher Gleason score are more likely to live long enough to have symptoms and disease progression in their lifetime and are better suited to more definitive treatment if the cancer is identified early at a low stage. The AUA recommends observation or watchful waiting for men with a life expectancy of 5 years or less with low-risk, localized prostate cancer.

Two large ongoing clinical trials are designed to compare watchful waiting with radical prostatectomy in men with clinically localized prostate cancer. The trial in the United States is the U.S. Prostate Cancer Intervention Versus Observation Trial (PIVOT) which compared radical prostatectomy to observation in men with localized prostate cancer over 19.5 years of follow-up (median of 12.7 years) found that in men with localized prostate cancer, surgery was not associated with lower all-cause or prostate cause mortality (*New England Journal of Medicine* 2017; 377: 132-140).

Pros and Cons of Watchful Waiting

There are several benefits to watchful waiting. **Morbidity**, meaning unhealthy results and complications of active treatment (e.g., incontinence, erectile dysfunction), is significant, especially in younger men. Risk of cancer progression with low-grade, low-stage tumor is low (10–25%) within 10 years. Rarely does low-grade, low-stage disease advance within 5 years.

On the downside, in men with nonmetastatic disease who survive more than 10 years, 63% die of prostate cancer. In younger patients with initially confined disease who undergo watchful waiting, there is a higher risk of developing incurable disease and dying from it.

Active Surveillance

Active surveillance is different than watchful waiting. It is based on the premise that some, but not all, patients may benefit from treatment of their cancer. Active surveillance involves actively monitoring the course of the disease with the expectation to intervene with curative intent if the cancer progresses.

There are two goals of active surveillance: (1) to provide definitive treatment for men with prostate cancer who are likely to progress, and (2) to decrease the risk of treatment-related complications for men with prostate cancer that is not likely to progress. The new AUA/ASTRO guidelines (www.auanet.org/guidelines) recommend active surveillance as the best available care option for very low-risk patients with localized prostate cancer. The guidelines also note that active surveillance is the preferred care option for most low-risk localized prostate cancer patients. It is not recommended for men with higher risk prostate cancer.

Morbidity
Unhealthy results and complications resulting from treatment.

Candidates for active surveillance are those individuals with lower-risk tumors (i.e., low Gleason score, low PSA, and low clinical stage). In addition, active surveillance is well suited for men with a shorter life expectancy. Active surveillance is appropriate for men with very low-risk prostate cancer when life expectancy is < 20 years or in men with low-risk prostate cancer when life expectancy is < 10 years. Some men with a longer life expectancy may be considered for active surveillance if they had very small areas of cancer in their biopsy or if they refuse other alternatives. However, if there is evidence of tumor progression while the patient has reasonable life expectancy, definitive treatment may be indicated.

The National Comprehensive Cancer Network (NCCN) guidelines recommend that follow-up on active surveillance should include:

- PSA no more often than every 6 months unless clinically indicated.
- DRE no more often than every 12 months unless clinically indicated.
- Needle biopsy of the prostate should be repeated within 6 months of diagnosis if initial biopsy consisted of fewer than 10 cores or was assessment discordant (i.e., palpable tumor contralateral to side of the biopsy).
- Needle biopsy should be considered as often as annually to assess for disease progression.
- Repeat biopsies not indicated when life expectancy is < 10 years or when men are on watchful waiting/observation.
- PSA doubling time appears unreliable for identification of progressive disease remains curable. Progression has occurred if Gleason score 4 or 5

found on repeat biopsy, and/or is found in greater number of biopsies, or occupies a greater extent of prostate biopsies.

The downsides of active surveillance include the risk that the patient will miss the opportunity for cure, the likelihood that nerve sparing surgery may be more difficult if the patient waits to have it, and the frequent doctor visits, lab tests, and biopsies that are involved.

The role of biomarker tests in active surveillance is unclear; currently the AUA/ASTRO guidelines indicate that tissue-based biomarkers have not shown a clear role in active surveillance for localized prostate cancer and therefore are not necessary.

84. Are there radioactive therapies for prostate cancer that, in addition to treating painful bone metastases, may help shrink my prostate cancer?

For men with significant bone pain and more extensive bone metastases, intravenous radionuclide treatments directed to bone metastases can be helpful. The FDA has approved several agents (see Question 90). More recently, radium 223 has been approved by the FDA for men with symptomatic bone metastases, with no known visceral metastases (Table 10, pages 148–152). It is administered intravenously every 4 weeks. **Radium 223** has been demonstrated to delay skeletal-related adverse events and increase overall survival (3.6 months) as well as decrease pain, coupled with a lower risk of a drop in the white blood cell and platelet counts compared to previously used therapies and thus is approved as a therapy

Radium 223

A radioisotope administered intravenously for the treatment of bone metastases.

for the treatment of symptomatic mCRPC. Monitoring of the white blood cell count is recommended during therapy. Other side effects include diarrhea, nausea, and vomiting.

Alternative medicine

The treatment is used instead of accepted treatments.

Acupuncture

A Chinese therapy involving the use of thin needles inserted into specific locations in the skin.

The most commonly used alternative therapies are acupuncture, biofeedback, chiropractic, energy healing, herbal medicine, homeopathy, hypnosis, imagery, massage, relaxation techniques, and vitamins and minerals.

85. What alternative therapies are available for prostate cancer?

Alternative medicine, or treatment that is different from accepted therapies, is commonly used in the United States, where more visits are made to alternative health providers than to primary care providers.

The most commonly used alternative therapies are acupuncture, biofeedback, chiropractic, energy healing, herbal medicine, homeopathy, hypnosis, imagery, massage, relaxation techniques, and vitamins and minerals.

Acupuncture is based on the belief that pathways of energy flow through the body that are essential for health and that changes in this flow can cause disease or illness. An acupuncturist uses needles to redirect or correct inadequate energy flow. On a more scientific basis, it appears that the placement of the needle in a certain location causes the release of chemicals from nerves that may alter one's perception of pain or cause the release of other chemicals that may affect perception of pain and may also improve healing. The National Institutes of Health have approved the use of acupuncture for relief of postoperative pain and treatment of nausea associated with chemotherapy. Its use in advanced-stage prostate cancer has possible advantages and disadvantages:

Advantages

- It may help relieve cancer-related pain.
- It may help relieve chemotherapy-induced nausea.
- It may affect the **immune response** (the response of organs, tissues, blood cells, and substances that fight off infections, cancers, or foreign substances) to cancer.
- It tends to promote more active management and involvement by the patient in his treatment.
- It may be covered by some managed care and insurance companies.
- Side effects are minimal if the acupuncturist is well trained.

Disadvantages

- Limited studies are available comparing a **placebo** (a fake medication or treatment that has no effect on the body) with acupuncture.
- No specific studies are available regarding the use of acupuncture in advanced prostate cancer.
- The patient needs to assess whether the acupuncturist is well trained because there are no specific training requirements in most states.
- If the acupuncturist is inexperienced, there is a risk of infection and injury.

If you are interested in acupuncture as a therapy for nausea, consult with your doctor—he or she might have a list of approved practitioners in your area. If not, the American Academy of Medical Acupuncture (AAMA) keeps a list of accredited practitioners nationwide, knows the laws governing the practice for your state, and has information regarding how acupuncture should be used. Contact information for the AAMA can be found in the **Appendix**.

Immune response

The response of organs, tissues, blood cells, and substances that fight off infections, cancers, or foreign substances.

Placebo

A fake medication ("candy pill") or treatment that has no effect on the body that is often used in experimental studies to determine if the experimental medication/treatment has an effect.

TREATMENT OF PROSTATE CANCER

Dietary Therapies

Lycopene is a carotenoid that is found in tomatoes and is a strong antioxidant. It may decrease the risk of prostate cancer. Several small studies have suggested a role for lycopene supplementation in men with prostate cancer; however, further studies are needed to determine whether or not it is truly effective.

Soy products are high in isoflavones, which have been shown to prevent cancer cell growth. The effects of soy supplementation in both prostate cancer prevention and in men with prostate cancer are being studied.

Herbal Remedies

It is important to note that herbal remedies sometimes have interactions with other medications or treatments, so you should never begin taking them without first consulting with your doctor. Herbal preparations are not monitored for purity by the FDA, so be cautious about what you buy; check the information on the label, and investigate the brands' reputations before you choose one.

86. When can I consider myself cured of prostate cancer?

Prostate cancer, like all cancers, does not "play by the rules." It does not reach out to areas outside of the prostate in a straight line such that if no cancer is present at the edge of the prostate then no cancer exists at all outside of the prostate. Cancer cells may remain in the pelvis, get into the bloodstream, or be present in the bones and not grow quickly enough for them to be noticed for several years. In the strictest sense, a cancer is considered to be "cured" when there is no evidence of any cancer 10 years after treatment. This seems like an awfully long time, and certainly you do not need to hold your breath and put your life on hold during this time; the PSA testing along the way will help assure you that all is going well. PSA testing is the most sensitive way of detecting a recurrence of the prostate cancer and detects it sooner than bone scans or other types of X-ray studies. With radical prostatectomy, the PSA decreases to an undetectable level in most people because the producer of PSA, the prostate, has been removed. Rarely, small glands in the urethra may produce very small amounts of PSA, which may account for a PSA level that is slightly above undetectable but does not increase over time. With radiation therapy, both interstitial seeds and EBRT, the prostate is not removed, and thus the PSA does not decrease to an undetectable range. The PSA will drop, however, reflecting the death of the cancer cells and the loss of PSA production. It should drop to ~0.5 ng/dL and remain at that level thereafter. Biopsy of the prostate is not routinely used to confirm that treatment has been effective after interstitial seed therapy or EBRT, because the changes that occur in the cells after radiation therapy make interpretation of the biopsy very difficult. The PSA is more helpful in this situation.

PART SIX

Complications of Treatment

Are there any predictors of recurrence of prostate cancer after "curative" therapy?

What happens if the PSA is rising after radiation therapy or radical prostatectomy?

My doctor has recommended that I be involved in a clinical trial. What is a clinical trial?

More . . .

87. Are there any predictors of recurrence of prostate cancer after "curative" therapy?

If one undergoes a radical prostatectomy, the surgical margins, the Gleason score, and the preoperative and postoperative PSA are good predictors of the likelihood of recurrence. The higher the preoperative prostate biopsy Gleason score (7 and higher) and PSA (> 20 ng/mL), the higher the likelihood of prostate cancer progression after surgery. For patients with prostate cancer that is pathologically confined to the prostate, the likelihood of being prostate cancer free as determined by PSA level is >90%. A Gleason score of the prostate specimen of 8 or higher is associated with an increased risk of prostate cancer progression. A researcher at Stanford University looked at the percent of high-grade cancer in the prostate specimen and found that the higher the percent of Gleason grade 4 or 5 in the tumor, the higher the risk of a rising postoperative PSA. The Gleason score and the initial PSA are also predictors of success of EBRT and interstitial seed therapy.

Several biomarkers may have a role in the determination of risk of recurrence of prostate cancer after definitive treatment (see Question 48). Decipher is a 22-gene test that determines a patient's probability of biochemical recurrence within 3 years or clinical metastatic disease from 5 to 10 years after radical prostatectomy. **ELAVL1** staining has been shown to be strongly associated with high Gleason grade, advanced tumor stage, positive lymph nodes, and PSA recurrence.

ELAVL1

RNA binding protein that may have a role in prostate cancer progression.

88. What happens if the PSA is rising after radiation therapy or radical prostatectomy?

After a radical prostatectomy, your PSA should decrease to an undetectable level (< 0.02 ng/mL, usually) by approximately 4 weeks post surgery. However, a detectable PSA level after this time does not mean that there is necessarily clinically significant recurrent prostate cancer. Some patients with a detectable PSA after radical prostatectomy do not have progression of their cancer because the PSA level is the result of the presence of benign prostate tissue at the margins of the resection (a very small amount of benign prostate tissue being left behind) or from a dormant residual focus of prostate cancer at a local or distant site. The definition of biochemical recurrence (evidence of recurrent prostate cancer based on PSA testing only) varies from a PSA of 0.2 ng/mL to 0.4 ng/mL post-radical prostatectomy. In a large number of patients, a biochemical recurrence of 0.2 ng/mL is associated with a slowly progressive course.

Your doctor will look at a variety of factors to determine if the rising PSA is due to benign tissue left behind at the time of surgery, locally recurrent prostate cancer that is amenable to radiation therapy, or metastatic prostate cancer that will require hormone therapy. Several investigators have looked at various criteria that may help distinguish local recurrence from distant metastases for patients with a rising PSA after radical prostatectomy. A Gleason score 8–10, seminal vesicle invasion, positive lymph nodes, and a rapid PSA velocity (rate of change of the PSA), and a short disease-free interval after radical prostatectomy have been associated with a greater chance of metastatic disease. Your doctor may also order a bone scan (see Question 43), a CT scan of the abdomen/pelvis, or PET CT (see Question 45).

Overall, about 35% of men who have had a radical prostatectomy will experience a detectable serum PSA within 10 years after surgery. The risk of developing metastatic disease after biochemical recurrence correlates with pathologic Gleason scores. Men with tumors of Gleason score < 8 have a 73% chance of remaining free of progression at 5 years after biochemical recurrence, compared with a < 10% probability in men with high-grade tumors (Gleason 8–10). The length of time after surgery prior to biochemical recurrence was important in determining the risk of eventual distant failure for men with lower (5–7) and men with higher (8–10) Gleason scores. Using a cutoff of 10 months, the prostate-specific antigen doubling time (PSADT) provides further substratification for men with Gleason scores of < 8. Men with a rapid rise in PSA (shorter PSA doubling time) have a greater risk of metastatic disease.

Several options are available, including watchful waiting, salvage EBRT, and hormone therapy.

Watchful Waiting

In one study, watchful waiting was used in men with a rising PSA after radical prostatectomy, and they were monitored until they had evidence of metastases. About 8 years after the radical prostatectomy, these men developed metastases, and an additional 5 years later, they died from their prostate cancer. In general, when watchful waiting is used for PSA progression after radical prostatectomy, the PSA is checked every 3 to 6 months to determine how quickly the PSA is rising (PSA velocity). If the **doubling time**, the time that it takes for the PSA level to double, is long (a year or longer), then

Doubling time

The amount of time that it takes for the PSA level to double.

the tumor is slow growing. If the doubling time is short (every 3 months), then the tumor is fast growing, and the patient would probably benefit from early treatment as opposed to continuing with watchful waiting.

Salvage Radiation Therapy

In males with a rising PSA after radical prostatectomy in whom the disease is felt to be locally recurrent, rather than metastatic, salvage radiation therapy is an option. The ASTRO consensus panel concluded that the appropriate PSA seemed to be 1.5 ng/mL for the institution of salvage radiation therapy. Others have demonstrated improved outcomes using a PSA threshold of 0.6. Gleason score 8–10, pre-radiotherapy PSA level > 2.0, negative surgical margin, PSA doubling time of 10 months or less, and seminal vesicle invasion are significant predictors of disease progression despite salvage radiation therapy. Conversely, a positive surgical margin suggests a greater likelihood that the recurrence is due to residual pelvic disease, therefore a patient with a history of a positive margin who develops an increasing PSA is most likely to benefit from salvage radiation therapy.

Hormone Therapy

Hormone therapy tends to be used more commonly for men with recurrent cancer in whom the recurrence is believed to be outside of the pelvic area. Although hormone therapy may delay the progression of the prostate cancer, its impact on survival in this situation is not well known. Men with high-grade tumors (Gleason sum > 7) or with cancer in the seminal vesicles or lymph nodes at the time of radical prostatectomy and in whom the PSA rises within 2 years after prostatectomy most likely have distant disease and are candidates for hormone therapy or watchful waiting.

Treatment of Rising PSA after EBRT

Historically, three consecutive PSA rises after achieving a PSA nadir was felt to be indicative of biochemical recurrence after EBRT. However, in 2005, a consensus panel meeting (RTOG-Astro Phoenix Consensus Conference) was held, which concluded that a PSA value of 2 ng/mL greater than the absolute nadir represents the best revised definition of failure following external-beam radiation monotherapy. In individuals with biochemical recurrence after EBRT, the options of treatment include salvage prostatectomy, salvage cryotherapy, hormone therapy, and watchful waiting. The decision regarding the most appropriate therapy is based on the likelihood of the cancer being confined to the prostate.

Salvage Prostatectomy After EBRT

The ideal patient for a salvage radical prostatectomy after EBRT is one who is believed to have had prostate-confined disease initially at the time of EBRT and who is still believed to have organ-confined disease. Individuals in this group include those who have a Gleason score ~6, a low pretreatment PSA level (< 10 ng/mL), and low clinical stage tumor (T1c or T2a). At the time of the salvage prostatectomy, they should still have a favorable Gleason score, a low clinical stage, and, ideally, a PSA that is < 4 ng/mL. Salvage prostatectomy is a challenging procedure, and if you are considering this option, you should seek out a urologist who has experience with it because there is an increased risk of urinary incontinence, erectile dysfunction, and rectal injury with this procedure. Rarely, because of extensive scarring, it is necessary to remove the bladder in addition to the prostate, and a urinary diversion would be necessary. A urinary diversion is a procedure that allows urine to be diverted to a segment of bowel that can be made into a storage unit similar to a bladder or allows urine to pass out of an opening in the belly wall into a bag, similar to a colostomy.

Salvage Cryotherapy

One of the main uses of cryotherapy is in patients with a rising PSA after EBRT. In patients who have not responded locally to EBRT, approximately 40% of the patients who then undergo salvage cryotherapy will have an undetectable PSA level after cryotherapy, and 78% will have negative prostate biopsy results. It appears that a drop in the PSA to ~0.5 ng/mL after cryotherapy is associated with a good prognosis. In men with post-cryotherapy PSA levels > 0.5 ng/mL, there is a higher likelihood that the PSA will increase or that the prostate biopsy result will be positive.

Hormone Therapy and Watchful Waiting

Use of these two options in patients with a rising PSA after EBRT is similar to their use in those with a rising PSA after radical prostatectomy.

Treatment of Rising PSA after Interstitial Seed Therapy

Treatment options for a rising PSA after interstitial seed therapy include salvage prostatectomy, EBRT, watchful waiting, and hormone therapy. It is important to remember that after interstitial seed therapy, there may be a benign rise in the PSA level, and this should not be misconstrued as being indicative of recurrent prostate cancer. In both interstitial seed and radiation therapy, for a rising PSA to be indicative of recurrent/ persistent prostate cancer, it must rise sequentially on three occasions at least 2 weeks apart. The treatment options are dependent on the likelihood of the disease being confined to the prostate. Salvage prostatectomy for interstitial seed failure carries the same risks as with EBRT failures. The ability to use EBRT depends on the amount of radiation that was delivered at the time of the interstitial seeds and the likelihood of the disease being confined to the prostate.

89. My doctor has recommended that I be involved in a clinical trial. What is a clinical trial?

Clinical trial

A carefully planned experiment to evaluate a treatment or medication (often a new drug) for an unproven use.

A **clinical trial** is a carefully planned experiment that is designed to evaluate the use of treatment or a medication for an unproven use. Through the use of clinical trials, investigators assess newer ideas in the treatment of various diseases. There are three different types of clinical trials, each with a particular goal. Typically, when a new medication or therapy is being introduced, its evaluation proceeds in an orderly process through each of these trials.

Phase I trials are preliminary, short-duration studies that involve only a few patients. These studies are used to see whether the medication or therapy has any effect or any serious side effects. *Phase II* trials involve a larger number of patients and are designed to determine the most active dose of the therapy as well as its side effects. *Phase III* trials involve large numbers of patients and compare the new therapy with the current standard or the best available therapy.

90. What treatment options are available if I have cancer in my bones?

When prostate cancer metastasizes, it tends to travel to the pelvic lymph nodes first and then to the bones. Bone metastases may be silent, meaning that they do not cause any pain, or they may be symptomatic, causing pain or leading to a fracture. Bone metastases are typically identified on a bone scan and can also be seen on a plain X-ray.

If you have not already tried hormone therapy (ADT) your doctor will start ADT as this can shrink the tumor deposits in your bone. If you develop bone metastases while on homone therapy, your doctor will try other forms of treatment for metastatic castrate-resistant prostate cancer (mCRPC). There are many ways to treat bone pain. Your doctor will likely try the simplest treatments and those associated with the least side effects first, and then progress as needed. Nonsteroidal anti-inflammatories such as ibuprofen (Advil) are typically used as a first-line treatment. If the pain is not controlled with these, then narcotics are added. For patients with a localized bone metastasis that is causing persistent discomfort, localized external-beam radiation (EBRT) to the bone may be used. EBRT is not used for men with multiple symptomatic bone metastases. EBRT provides pain relief in 80% to 90% of patients, and the relief may last for some time. Usually, the total dose of radiation is given over 1 to 2 weeks' duration. The side effects of the localized EBRT vary with the area that is being irradiated. Treatment of metastases to the skull may cause hair loss and flaking and redness of the scalp. Treatment of cervical spine (neck bone) metastases may cause discomfort with swallowing and hoarseness. If the mid-spine is treated, nausea and vomiting may result.

Treatment of pelvic bone metastases may cause diarrhea. Treatment side effects often resolve with time.

When multiple painful bone metastases are present, hemibody radiation may be used. Because this therapy affects a larger area of the body, there are more side effects, including lowering of the blood pressure (hypotension), nausea, vomiting, diarrhea, lung irritation, hair loss, and lowering of the blood count. **Hemibody** radiation is also given over several treatment sessions. It can lead to pain control that lasts up to a year for as many as 70% of individuals.

Hemibody

Half of the body.

Another form of therapy for multiple painful bone metastases is radioisotope therapy. With this form of therapy, a radioisotope is attached to a chemical that is actively picked up by the bones and injected into a vein. The radioactively labeled chemical is picked up by the bone and "radiates" the area. Historically, strontium 89 and samarium 153 were the more commonly used isotopes. Their use improved bone pain in 80% to 86% of individuals, however, they were associated with the lowering of the white blood cell count, which limited retreatment rates. They also did not appear to have a significant effect on survival. A new radioisotope, radium 223 (Xotigo) has been approved which has fewer effects on the white blood cell count. It has been demonstrated to not only improve pain, but also to increase survival by several months. It is approved for men with symptomatic mCRPC without visceral metastases (see Question 84).

RANK-ligand inhibitor

A chemical that binds that prevents RANK-ligand from functioning.

Other therapies including the bisphosphonate zoledronic acid (Zometa) and the **RANK-ligand inhibitor** denosumab (Prolia, Xgeva), are used in men with bone metastases to decrease the risk of skeletal-related adverse events (bone fracture).

Zoledronic acid is administered by an intravenous infusion that takes about 15 minutes and is given every 3 to 4 weeks. You will need to have your kidney function checked before each administration. It is recommended that you continue your calcium and vitamin D supplementation in addition to the infusion. Side effects include nausea, fatigue, anemia, bone pain, constipation, fever, vomiting, and shortness of breath. A less common side effect of zoledronic acid and other bisphosphonates is **osteonecrosis of the jaw** (**ONJ**). ONJ is an uncommon but severe side effect of bisphosphonate drugs. It can occur following dental surgery, such as having a tooth removed. A sign of ONJ is poor healing of an area of bone exposed after dental surgery. There might or might not be pain, swelling, infection, or drainage associated with ONJ. Treatment of ONJ will vary with severity. Unhealthy bone may need to be removed, and any associated infections should be treated. Rinsing your mouth with antibacterial mouth rinses help prevent infections, and treatment with the **bisphosphonate** should be stopped. There appears to be some improvement in ONJ at least 6 months after stopping treatment with the bisphosphonate.

Because of these potential complications, it is recommended that the patient maintain good mouth hygiene and should have a dental examination with preventive dentistry prior to starting bisphosphonates. You should also inform your dentist prior to starting a bisphosphonate so that any necessary dental procedures can be performed before your bisphosphonate therapy starts. Ideally, you should avoid any invasive dental procedures while on a bisphosphonate. If you need an invasive dental procedure while on a bisphosphonate, it is unclear whether stopping the bisphosphonate decreases the risk of ONJ.

Osteonecrosis of the jaw (ONJ)

A severe bone disease that affects the bones of the jaw, maxilla, and mandible. It may occur in association with bisphosphonate and RANK-ligand inhibitor use.

Biphosphonate

A type of medication that is used to treat osteoporosis and the bone pain caused by some types of cancer.

Denosumab is a RANK-ligand inhibitor. Our bones are continuously being remodeled. Old bone tissue is removed and replaced with new bone tissue. The cells that break down bone are called **osteoclasts**. The body (bone) does not make osteoclast cells; rather, osteoclasts develop from precursor cells, "pre-osteoclasts." These "pre-osteoclasts" are stimulated to develop into osteoclasts by the attachment of a special molecule, cytokine RANK-ligand, a specialized area on the cell, the RANK-ligand receptor. Denosumab is an antibody that attaches to the RANK-ligand receptor, thus preventing the "pre-osteoclast" from developing into an osteoclast. Denosumab is administered by intramuscular injection once every 4 weeks. Because it is associated with the lowering of the calcium level, it is important that one takes calcium and vitamin D when receiving denosumab. Compared to placebo, denosumab was associated with a lower incidence of bone fractures in men with bone metastases, 1.5% compared to 3.9% with placebo. The most common side effects include the lowering of the calcium level, urinary tract infection, lower respiratory tract infection (i.e., lung infection), cataracts, constipation, rashes, eczema, and joint pain. Although it is not a bisphosphonate, denosumab use could increase the risk of ONJ and thus, the same guidelines should be followed.

When compared to zoledronic acid, denosumab 120 mg (Xgeva) has been demonstrated to delay the time to the first skeletal-related event and significantly reduce the first and subsequent skeletal-related events compared to zoledronic acid in men with prostate cancer and bone metastases.

Osteoclast

A specialized cell that breaks down bone.

91. What is erectile dysfunction (ED), and what happens if I have ED after treatment for my prostate cancer?

Cliff's comment:

When I was told that there were two major long-term risks of surgery, loss of control of urine and erectile dysfunction, I can remember thinking that I can live with impotence but please God, don't let me be incontinent of urine. Well, I underwent a unilateral nerve-sparing prostatectomy, and although I do not get spontaneous erections on my own, I am happy that the "little blue pill"—Viagra—works. "Does it give you the same strength and endurance that you had years ago?" you may ask. I ask, "Does anything you do in your 60s have the same strength and endurance it had years ago?" I am very happy with the oral therapy, and it has remedied my erectile troubles.

Erectile dysfunction is the consistent inability to achieve adequate penile rigidity for penetration or adequate duration of rigidity for completion of sexual performance. Approximately 50% of men 40 to 70 years of age experience erectile dysfunction. To achieve an adequate erection, you must have properly functioning nerves, arteries, and veins. When you are stimulated or aroused, your brain releases chemicals that tell the nerves in the pelvis to release chemicals that in turn tell the arteries in the penis to open and increase blood flow into the penis. At the same time that blood is moving into the penis, the veins in the penis collapse so that the blood remains in the penis, making it rigid and allowing the rigidity to last. Anything that can affect the brain, nerves, arteries, or veins can cause trouble with erections. More common causes of erectile dysfunction include strokes; spinal cord injury; Parkinson's disease; high cholesterol levels; heart disease; poor circulation in the legs; high blood pressure and medications used to treat high blood pressure; depression and medications used to treat depression; diabetes; surgery, such as radical prostatectomy and colorectal cancer surgeries; pelvic radiation; and hormone therapy for prostate cancer.

When seeking treatment for prostate cancer, many men are very concerned about the effects of the treatment on erectile function. Basically, all of the treatment options carry a risk of erectile dysfunction; however, they differ in how soon after treatment the erectile dysfunction occurs and how likely it is to occur. If you are already having trouble with erections, none of the treatments for prostate cancer will improve your erections. The incidence of erectile dysfunction associated with radical prostatectomy varies with patient age, erectile function before surgery, nerve-sparing status, and the surgeon's technical ability to perform a nerve-sparing radical prostatectomy. The incidence of erectile dysfunction after a nerve-sparing radical prostatectomy varies from 16% to 82%. When it occurs with radical prostatectomy, erectile dysfunction is immediate and is related to the damage of the pelvic nerves, which travel along the outside edge of the prostate. Men who have undergone nerve-sparing radical prostatectomies who are impotent after surgery may experience return of their erectile function over the following 12 months.

The incidence of erectile dysfunction after EBRT ranges from 32% to 67% and is caused by radiation-related damage to the arteries. Unlike with surgery, the erectile dysfunction occurs a year or more after the radiation. The incidence of erectile dysfunction is 15% to 31% in the first year after EBRT and 40% to 62% at 5 years after EBRT.

The incidence of erectile dysfunction after interstitial seed therapy with or without medium-dose EBRT ranges from 6% to 50%. Similar to EBRT, the erectile dysfunction tends to occur later than with radical prostatectomy.

Hormone therapy with the GnRH agonists or orchiectomy also causes erectile dysfunction, as well as loss of interest in sex (libido) in most men. This loss of libido is related to the loss of testosterone, but why the loss of testosterone causes troubles with erections is not well known.

Various therapies are available for the treatment of erectile dysfunction, including oral, intraurethral, and injection therapies; the vacuum device; and the **penile prosthesis**, which is a device that is surgically placed into the penis that allows an impotent individual to have an erection (**Table 11**, pages 182–186). Oral therapies currently available include Viagra (sildenafil), Cialis (tadalafil), Levitra (vardenafil), and **Stendra (avanafil)**. They all work in a similar fashion to increase blood flow to the penis during sexual stimulation. Injection therapies include prostaglandin E1 (Caverjet, Edex) and Trimix, a combination of papaverine, phentolamine, and prostaglandin E1. Injection therapies do not require sexual stimulation to be effective. Nerve grafting, whereby a nerve is removed from another area of the body and sewn into the site where the pelvic nerve was removed, is being evaluated.

Penile prosthesis

A device that is surgically placed into the penis which allows an impotent individual to have an erection.

Stendra (avanafil)

A phosphodiesterase type V inhibitor used to treat erectile dysfunction.

In the treatment of post–radical prostatectomy erectile dysfunction, the effectiveness of Viagra and other medications like it (Levitra, Cialis, Stendra) varies with nerve-sparing status:

- Bilateral nerve sparing: 71% success rate
- Unilateral nerve sparing: 50% success rate
- Non–nerve sparing: 15% success rate

Table 11 Treatment Options for Erectile Dysfunction

Rx	Administration	Dosing	Success Rate	Contraindications	Side Effects	Mechanisms of Action
Sildenafil (Viagra)	Oral: taken on demand 0.5–1.5 hr before intercourse, requires stimulation.	25, 50, 100 mg, lower dose if > 65 yr, use newer protease inhibitors, erythromycin, ketoconazole with hepatic/renal failure; 78% pts prefer 100 mg. Use only once per 24 hr.	48–81%; varies with etiology of erectile dysfunction.	Concomitant nitrate use, retinitis pigmentosa. When using concomitant alpha-blockers, patient should be on stable dose of alpha-blocker prior to starting Viagra; start with 25 mg. Follow Princeton guidelines regarding use in CV pts.	HA in 16%, flushing in 10%, dyspepsia in 7%, visual disturbance in 3%, priapism uncommon. NAION (nonarteritic anterior ischemic optic neuropathy) has been reported in individuals taking PDE 5 inhibitors, but a causal relationship has not been identified. The risk factors for NAION are similar to those for ED, such as age > 50 yr, HT, increased cholesterol, and DM. Another risk factor is a small cup-to-disk ratio. Pts should be advised to seek medical attention in the event of a sudden loss of vision in one or both eyes. Hearing loss has also been reported in patients taking PDE5 inhibitors. As with NAION a causal relationship has not been established.	Phosphodiesterase type V inhibitor leads to increased cGMP, which stimulates cavernous small muscle relaxation.

Rx	Administration	Dosing	Success Rate	Contraindications	Side Effects	Mechanisms of Action
Tadalafil (Cialis)	Oral—taken on demand 2 hr before intercourse, requires stimulation.	Daily dosing now available. 5 mg, 10 mg, 20 mg. Recommended starting dose in most pts is 10 mg. Start at 5 mg if moderate renal insufficiency, lower dose if on CYP3A4 inhibitors. Cialis has a long half-life of 17–21 hr, which may provide for efficacy for up to 36 hr, however, may be taken once every 24 hr. 2.5 mg once daily approved.	62–77% success with penetration (SEP 2) and 50–64% success with maintaining erection (SEP 3).	Nitrates, retinitis pigmentosa; if using alpha-blockers, must be stable on alpha-blocker therapy and start with lowest dose if Cialis. Follow Princeton guidelines regarding use in CV pts.	HA 11–15%, dyspepsia 4–10%, myalgia 1–3%, back pain 3–6%, flushing 2–3%. NAION—see Sildenafil side effects. Hearing loss—see Sildenafil side effects.	Phosphodiesterase type V inhibitor leads to increased cGMP, which stimulates cavernous small muscle relaxation.

(continues)

Table 11 Treatment Options for Erectile Dysfunction (continued)

Rx	Administration	Dosing	Success Rate	Contraindications	Side Effects	Mechanisms of Action
Vardenafil (Levitra)	Oral—taken on demand 25 minutes to 60 minutes before intercourse, requires stimulation.	2.5 mg, 5 mg, 10 mg, 20 mg. Recommended starting dose in most pts is 10 mg. Start at 5 mg in pts ≥ 65 yr, lower doses when concomitant use with CYP3A4 inhibitors.	Improvements in SEP 2 (ability to penetrate) of 75–80% (10–20 mg) compared to 52% with placebo and maintenance of erection SEP 3 of 64–65% (10–20 mg) compared to 32% placebo.	Nitrates, retinitis pigmentosa; if using alpha-blockers, must be stable on alpha-blocker therapy and start with lowest dose of vardenafil. Follow Princeton guidelines regarding use in cardiovascular pts. May increase QTc interval and thus avoid use in individuals with congenital QT prolongation and those taking Class IA or III anti-arrhythmics.	HA 15%, flushing 11%, dyspepsia 4%. NAION—See Sildenafil side effects. Hearing loss—see Sildenafil side effects.	Phosphodiesterase type V inhibitor leads to increased cGMP, which stimulates cavernous small muscle relaxation.
Avanafil (Stendra)	Oral: take on demand 15 minutes prior to intercourse.	50 mg, 100 mg, 200 mg. Use once per 24 hrs. Starting dose 100 mg; 50 mg if on concomitant alpha blocker.	46–74% success rate.	Concomitant use of nitrates. Concomitant use of guanylate cyclase stimulator; prior history of hypersensitivity	Headache 5.1–10.5% Flushing 3.2–4.0% Nasal congestion 1.8–2.0% Nasopharyngitis 0.9–3.4% Back pain 3.2–1.1%	Phosphodiesterase type V inhibitor leads to increased cGMP, which stimulates cavernous smooth muscle relaxation.

Rx	Administration	Dosing	Success Rate	Contraindications	Side Effects	Mechanisms of Action
Avanafil (Stendra) (continued)				reaction; same concerns with concomitant alpha blockers as other PDE V inhibitors.	Same risks of NAION and hearing loss as other PDE V inhibitors.	
Intraurethral alprostadil	Small suppository placed into distal urethra via small applicator.	125, 250, 500, 1000 μg. Use only once per 24 hr.	30–66% success rate (N Engl J Med 1997; 336:1).	Hypersensitivity to PGE1, pregnant partner, predisposition to priapism (leukemia, multiple myeloma, sickle cell).	Pain (penile, urethral, testicular, perineal) in 33%, lowers blood pressure in 3%, priapism, vaginal irritation in 10%.	Absorbed through urethral mucosa and stimulates arterial dilation and flow.
Intracavernous injection therapy with alprostadil	Direct injection into lateral aspect of corpora cavernosa, alternating sides with each injection.	5 μg to > 40 μg; dose depends on etiology of ED; test dose at 10 μg; if suspect neurologic disease, use 5-μg test dose; use only once per 48–72 hr.	Average success rate 73% (Int J Impot Res 1994;6:149; J Urol 1988; 140:66).	Known hypersensitivity to alprostadil. Pts at risk for priapism. Pts at increased risk: those on anticoagulants and with Peyronie's disease.	Prolonged erections in 1.1–1.3%, corporal fibrosis in 2.7%, painful erection in 15–30%, hematoma, ecchymosis in 1.5%.	Alprostadil stimulates cavernous small muscle relaxation, causes modulation of adenyl cyclase, increase in cAMP and subsequent free Ca²⁺ conc.

(continues)

Table 11 Treatment Options for Erectile Dysfunction (continued)

Rx	Administration	Dosing	Success Rate	Contraindications	Side Effects	Mechanisms of Action
Vacuum constriction device	Plastic cylinder with hand- or battery-operated pump and constricting bands.	N/A. Remove band within 30 min after application.	68–83% satisfaction rate.	Painful ejaculation: 3–16%, inability to ejaculate: 12–30%, petechiae of penis: 25–39%, numbness during erection: 5% (J Urol 1993;149:290; Spahn M, Manning M, Juenemann KP. Textbook of Erectile Dysfunction) Carson C, Kirby R, Goldstein I. Oxford: Isis Medical Media 1999. Intracavernosal therapy.	Use with caution in pts taking aspirin or anticoagulants.	Vacuum device creates negative pressure that pulls blood into corpora cavernosa; constriction band prolongs erection by decreasing corporal venous drainage.
Penile prosthesis	Surgically placed, models range from semirigid to inflatable.	N/A	> 90% satisfaction with inflatable prostheses (J Urol 1993; 150:1814; 1992;147:62).	Decreases penile length by 1 cm. Infection < 10%, diabetics at increased risk. Mechanical malfunction < 5% (Urol Clin North Am 1995;22:847). Erosion: increased risk in diabetics and spinal cord injury pts.	Requires counseling, preoperative.	Cylinders placed in corpora cavernosa provide penile rigidity; once placed, there is corporal fibrosis; if removed, remaining options less likely to work.

Reprinted with permission from Ellsworth P, Rous SN, Onion DK (ed.). *Blackwell's Primary Care Essentials: Urology*. West Sussex, UK: John Wiley & Sons, Ltd., 2001.

Most men with post–radical prostatectomy erectile dysfunction require 100 mg of Viagra to achieve an erection. In men with EBRT-associated erectile dysfunction, Viagra works in about 71%. Lastly, in men who have erectile dysfunction associated with interstitial seed therapy, Viagra has a success rate of approximately 80%. There are four oral medications currently available for erectile dysfunction: Viagra, Levitra, Cialis, and Stendra. All of these medications are effective in treating erectile dysfunction. All of these require sexual stimulation/foreplay and functioning pelvic nerves for it to be effective. It prevents the breakdown of chemicals released by the pelvic nerves; thus, there is more chemical around to tell the arteries in the penis to open up. To be effective, they must be taken about 30 minutes to 1 hour (2 hours for Cialis) before sexual stimulation. A daily dosing of Cialis is now available, which does not require taking at a specified time before intercourse, as long as one is taking it on a daily basis. When you take Viagra or Stendra, you should avoid a high-fat meal around the time of its use because this would prevent the medication from working as well; one does not have to avoid a high-fat meal when taking Levitra. Cialis has a longer half-life than the other three drugs, and in some men may provide the ability to have an erection a day or two after taking the medication (Table 11, pages 182–186).

Viagra, Levitra, Stendra, and Cialis are not for everyone, and you should consult with your doctor before taking any of these medications. Men with unstable angina who use nitroglycerin on a daily or frequent basis should not take any of these medications, nor should men with poorly functioning hearts (congestive heart failure) or men who have high blood pressure that requires several medications to control.

Another drug that is used to treat erectile dysfunction is intraurethral alprostadil (Muse), a small pellet that comes preloaded in an applicator (**Figure 17**, page 188). To use Muse, you should void first to lubricate the urethra with urine before you insert the applicator. Other lubricants, such as K-Y Jelly® and Vaseline®, cannot be used for this purpose. The applicator is placed into the tip of the penis, and the small button at the other end is pressed (**Figure 18**, page 189), thus releasing a small suppository. Gentle rubbing of the penis dissolves the suppository in the urethra, and the medication is absorbed. The most common side effect of Muse is urethral/penile burning or pain, and men who have undergone a radical prostatectomy seem to have an increased incidence of this side effect. Muse works in 20% to 40% of men with post–radical prostatectomy erectile dysfunction and has a similar success rate for post-EBRT erectile dysfunction.

The vacuum device is composed of several parts: a plastic tube that has a constricting band loaded on it and a pump, either hand-held or battery-operated (**Figure 19**, page 189) The plastic tube with the preloaded constricting band is placed over the lubricated penis. The pump is then

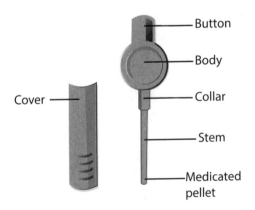

Figure 17 Intraurethral alprostadil (Muse).
Reproduced with permission from Meda Pharmaceuticals, Somerset, New Jersey.

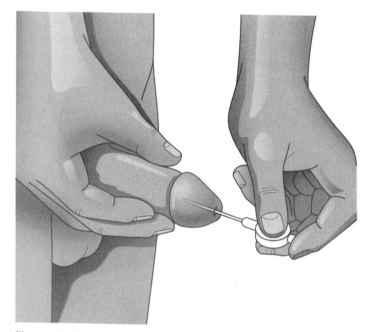

Figure 18 Muse insertion.
Data from © 2002 Krames StayWell.

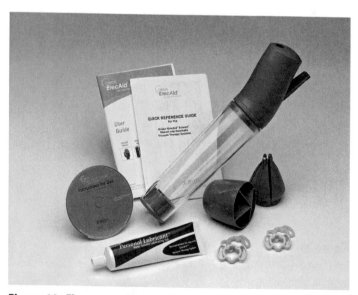

Figure 19 The vacuum device.
Courtesy of ErecAid.

activated, causing a suction that pulls blood into the penis. When the penis is rigid, the constricting band is pulled off of the tube so that it is positioned around the base of the penis; this band serves to hold the blood in the penis. When intercourse is completed, the band is removed, and the blood drains out of the penis. The band should be removed within 30 minutes after placement to prevent damage to the penis. The band may affect the ability to ejaculate, but won't affect the orgasm (ability to climax). In men who have had a radical prostatectomy, there will be no fluid (ejaculate), at the time of orgasm. Men who have had EBRT or interstitial seed therapy still have an ejaculate, but the volume may be diminished.

Injection therapy sounds much more painful than it actually is. It involves using a very tiny needle and injecting a small amount of a fluid into the side of the penis (**Figure 20**, page 190). The most commonly used form of injection therapy is prostaglandin E1 (Caverject or

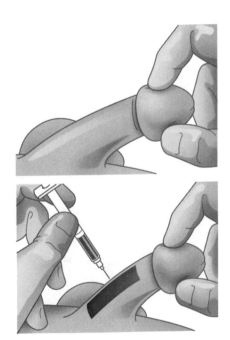

Figure 20
Injection therapy: proper location of injection.
Data from: Pharmacia-UpJohn/ Pfizer, Inc.

Edex). Approximately 30% of men experience discomfort with the prostaglandin E1; these individuals can try a combination therapy, such as triple P/Trimix (phentolamine, papaverine, and prostaglandin), which contains less prostaglandin. Trimix is associated with less pain but tends to cause more scarring in the penis than prostaglandin E1 alone. These chemicals tell the blood vessels to open up and increase blood flow into the penis. They work within 10 to 20 minutes after the injection and ideally produce an erection that lasts an hour or so.

Injection therapy works in more than 85% of men with post–radical prostatectomy erectile dysfunction. It may be used in men who have undergone nerve-sparing radical prostatectomies while they await the return of nerve function. In fact, some small studies suggest that early use of injection therapy after radical prostatectomy may quicken the recovery of nerve function. Injection therapy is also very successful in post–EBRT and post–seed placement erectile dysfunction. There is a small risk (2%) that the erection produced may last longer than 4 to 6 hours; this condition is called **priapism**. If you experience an erection that lasts longer than 3 to 4 hours, you should call the urologist on call because this condition needs to be treated immediately; otherwise, pain or damage to the penis could result, and the condition becomes more difficult to treat. If you seek help early, then all the doctor may have to do is inject another chemical into the penis to tell the blood vessels to shut down. When performing injection therapy, you should alternate sides of the penis and not perform the injections any more frequently than every 48 to 72 hours to prevent scar tissue from forming.

A penile prosthesis or implant is a permanent device that is placed into the penis. Several types of penile prostheses exist that vary in their complexity. There are semirigid

Priapism

An erection that lasts longer than 4 to 6 hours.

prostheses and inflatable prostheses. The semirigid prosthesis remains the same width at all times; you bend the penis up when you wish to have intercourse and down to conceal the penis. This prosthesis is the easiest to put in and has the least risk of mechanical malfunction, but it provides the least natural-looking result. Inflatable prostheses have the advantage of looking natural: in the deflated state, the penis is flaccid, and in the inflated state, the penis becomes erect. Two types of inflatable prostheses are available: a two piece and a three piece.

The two-piece unit is composed of two cylinders, one placed in each side of the penis, and a small pump that is placed in the scrotum. Squeezing the scrotal pump pushes fluid into the cylinders, distending them and making the penis erect. The three-piece unit has two cylinders, a scrotal pump, and a reservoir that sits under the abdominal wall near the bladder (**Figure 21**, page 192). The reservoir contains a larger amount of fluid, which allows for more rigidity than is possible with the two-piece unit.

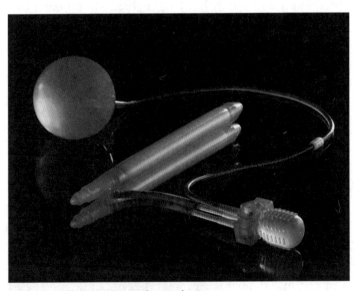

Figure 21 Three-piece penile prosthesis.
Courtesy of AMS - American Medical Systems, Inc.

As the complexity of the prostheses increases, so does the risk of mechanical trouble. Over the years, these devices have been revised such that the malfunction rate is about 10% at 10 years. One of the most distressing risks of placement of a penile prosthesis is infection. Although this risk is small, if the device becomes infected, the whole device must be removed and, in most cases, another device cannot be inserted at the same time. Once a prosthesis has been placed, other forms of treatment for erectile dysfunction usually do not work, although, occasionally, the vacuum device does work in men who have had the prosthesis removed. Thus, it is important to try other forms of therapy for erectile dysfunction and to make sure that they are either ineffective or that you do not like them before you proceed with a penile prosthesis. The satisfaction rate with a penile prosthesis is about 90% for both the man and his partner.

Sural nerve grafting is an investigational therapy for the treatment of erectile dysfunction related to non–nerve sparing radical prostatectomy. During a radical prostatectomy in which the neurovascular bundle(s) are removed, a segment of the sural nerve (a nerve located in the leg) is removed and is sewn into the place where the neurovascular bundle was. Preliminary results with this technique demonstrate that it can improve postoperative erectile dysfunction and that it may also allow for fewer positive margins because the surgeon is able to remove more tissue surrounding the prostate. However, it remains investigational.

A topical gel composed of prostaglandin E1 is being evaluated. This agent would be applied to the penis, and certain SEPAs, skin penetration enhancers, allows the prostaglandin to penetrate through the skin and pass into the corpora to increase penile blood flow.

Alprostadil cream (Vitaros) has been available to treat erectile dysfunction in the United Kingdom since June 2014. It is not currently available in the United States. It is a cream that when applied to the penis is absorbed through the skin and increases blood flow into the penis.

92. I am incontinent after my prostate cancer. What can I do?

Urinary incontinence, the uncontrolled loss of urine, is one of the most bothersome risks of prostate cancer treatment. Although it is more commonly associated with radical prostatectomy, it may also occur after interstitial seed therapy, EBRT, and cryotherapy. Urinary incontinence may lead to anxiety, hopelessness, and loss of self-control and self-esteem. Fear of leakage may limit social activities and participation in sex. If you are experiencing these feelings, you should discuss this with your doctor and spouse or significant other.

If you experience persistent urinary incontinence after surgery or radiation therapy, your doctor will want to identify the degree and the type of incontinence. You will be asked questions regarding the number of pads you use per day, what activities precipitate the incontinence, how frequently you urinate, if you have frequency or urgency, how strong your force of urine stream is, if you feel that you are emptying your bladder well, and what types and how much fluid you are drinking. The doctor may check to make sure that you are emptying your bladder well. This is usually done by having you urinate and then scanning your bladder with a small ultrasound probe to determine how much urine is left behind. Normally, less than 50 mL remains after urination.

Several different types of urinary incontinence exist, and the different types may coexist. The treatment of urinary incontinence varies with the type, and the types that may be encountered in men being treated for prostate cancer include stress, overflow, and urge incontinence. Men who have undergone radical prostatectomy typically experience a type of **stress incontinence** called "intrinsic sphincter deficiency." Stress incontinence may also occur after interstitial seed therapy and is much more common if a TURP of the prostate was performed in the past. In men, urinary control is primarily at the bladder outlet by the internal sphincter muscle. This muscle remains closed and opens only during urination. An additional muscle, the external sphincter, is located further away from the bladder and is the "backup" muscle. The external sphincter is the muscle that you contract when you feel the urge to urinate and there is no bathroom in sight. During a radical prostatectomy, the internal sphincter is often damaged with the removal of the prostate because it lies just at the top of the prostate. Continence then depends on the ability of the remaining urethra to close (**coapt**) and on the external sphincter.

Urge incontinence is the involuntary loss of urine associated with the urgency (a sudden, compelling desire to urinate that is difficult to defer) and is related to an overactive bladder. Although less common than intrinsic sphincter deficiency in men who have undergone radical prostatectomy, it may be present alone or in conjunction with intrinsic sphincter deficiency. Overactive bladder and decreased bladder capacity are more common in men who have undergone EBRT for prostate cancer.

Overflow incontinence is the involuntary loss of urine related to incomplete emptying of the bladder.

Stress incontinence

The involuntary loss of urine during sudden rises in intra-abdominal pressure, e.g., with coughing, laughing, sneezing, or picking up heavy objects.

Coapt

To close or fasten together.

Urge incontinence

The involuntary loss of urine associated with the urge to urinate and is related to an overactive bladder.

Overflow incontinence

The involuntary loss of urine related to incomplete emptying of the bladder.

COMPLICATIONS OF TREATMENT

After radical prostatectomy, this may occur if significant scarring (a bladder neck contracture) is present at the bladder outlet area. Treatment of the bladder neck contracture often relieves the overflow incontinence. Other symptoms include a weak urine stream and the feeling of incomplete bladder emptying. With overflow incontinence, the bladder scanner would demonstrate a large amount of urine left in the bladder after urinating. Urethral strictures after EBRT may also cause overflow incontinence; dilation of such strictures also improves the overflow incontinence. Urethral strictures tend to recur, and daily in-and-out passage of a catheter beyond the site of the stricture helps prevent recurrence of the stricture. Swelling of the prostate after interstitial seed therapy may cause voiding troubles, which if unrecognized, may lead to overflow incontinence. Initial treatment of overflow incontinence after seed therapy is with clean intermittent catheterization, and possibly the addition of an alpha-blocker (Hytrin, Cardura, Flomax, Rapaflo, Uroxatral) and a nonsteroidal anti-inflammatory.

Your responses to the questions your doctor asks regarding your incontinence will help your doctor determine the type and the severity of your urinary incontinence. To help determine the type(s) of urinary incontinence that you experience your doctor may recommend a fluoroscopic urodynamic study, which is a special study designed to measure the pressures in your bladder during voiding and at the time of urinary leakage (if it occurs during the study) and to look at the urethra and bladder during bladder filling and urinating. The study involves the placement of a catheter through the penis into the bladder. The catheter is connected to a pressure monitor, and sterile contrast fluid is run through the catheter into the bladder. Periodic X-ray studies are taken to determine whether the bladder outlet is open and if leakage is occurring. During the study, you will be asked to bear down as though you were trying to have a bowel movement, and you will be checked for leakage during this maneuver. Often, men with stress incontinence leak during the bearing down (Valsalva), and the bladder pressure at which this leakage occurs, the Valsalva leak point pressure, is an important predictor of the success of various treatment options. During the urodynamic study, an overactive bladder is identified by intermittent increases in bladder pressure during bladder filling that may be associated with leakage or the urge to urinate.

Treatment Options

Once the cause and the severity of the urinary incontinence has been assessed, you can then embark on treatment. In all cases of incontinence, it is important to make sure that you are voiding regularly, that is, every 3 hours, and avoiding alcohol and caffeinated fluids. Caffeine and alcohol cause the kidneys to make more urine and may also irritate the bladder. It may also be helpful to avoid acidic foods and foods with a lot of hot spices because these may also act as bladder irritants.

If a bladder neck contracture is present, treatment may consist of dilation or incision. There is a risk of stress incontinence after the incision of a bladder neck contracture. If overflow incontinence occurs after interstitial seed therapy, your doctor may give you a medication called an alpha-blocker (which relaxes the prostate) and an anti-inflammatory drug, and also prescribe clean intermittent catheterization until you are voiding on your own. Usually, voiding troubles of this nature after interstitial seed therapy resolve with time; rarely is additional treatment needed. Your doctor will be quite reluctant to do anything more aggressive for the first

6 months after the placement of the seeds because of the high risk of urinary incontinence with a TURP.

Overactive bladder is treated with medications that relax the bladder muscle, the most common of which are called anticholinergics, including oxybutynin (Ditropan), Ditropan XL, tolterodine (Detrol), Detrol LA, solifenacin (Vesicare), trospium chloride (Sanctura), Sanctura XR, darifenacin (Enablex), patch (Oxytrol) oxybutynin, and fesoterodine (Toviaz). Side effects of these medications include dry mouth, facial flushing, constipation, and blurry vision. These are decreased with the long-acting forms.

A variety of treatment options exist for stress incontinence, including pelvic floor muscle exercises, a penile clamp, collagen injection, an artificial sphincter, and a male urethral sling.

Pelvic floor muscle exercises

Exercises that help one strengthen muscles that aid in the control of urinary incontinence.

Pelvic floor muscle exercises: These exercises are intended to strengthen the pelvic floor muscles. To identify these muscles, simply try stopping your urine stream while you are urinating. Pelvic floor muscle exercises involve repetitive contracting and relaxing of the pelvic muscles at least 20 times per day every day of the week. Pelvic floor stimulation and biofeedback allow you to identify these muscles better and to monitor the strength of the contractions. These exercises are very helpful initially, when the catheter is removed after radical prostatectomy. They are not as effective in men who have undergone prior pelvic irradiation.

Penile clamp

A device placed around the penis to prevent urine leakage.

Penile clamp: Several penile clamps are available, and all of them have the same principle—to compress the urethra to prevent urinary leakage (**Figure 22**, page 199).

They should be worn for brief periods of time only and should not be left on all day. If they are left on for long periods of time, they may cause damage to the penile skin and the urethra. The clamp needs to be removed if you need to urinate. The penile clamp should not take the place of pelvic floor muscle exercises; rather, it should be used as a backup measure, for instance, if you are going out to dinner and want to make certain there is no leakage.

Collagen injection: Collagen is a chemical that is found throughout your body. The collagen that is being used to treat urinary incontinence is derived from a cow. Because it comes from a source outside of your body, you must have skin testing to make sure that you are not allergic to the collagen. Skin testing involves injecting a small amount of the collagen under your skin and then periodically inspecting the site, as one does with a PPD (tuberculosis) test. If the site becomes red and swollen, then you are allergic to the collagen and cannot undergo collagen injections. However, allergic reactions to collagen are very uncommon.

The collagen is injected into the bladder neck and the proximal urethra to make the urethra come together (coapt) (**Figure 23**, page 200). Often, more than one treatment session is needed; typically three to four injections,

Collagen injection

Injection of a chemical around the urethra that compresses the urethra and bladder neck to help treat stress urinary incontinence.

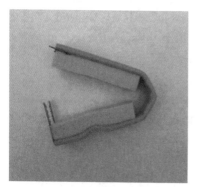

Figure 22
Penile clamp.

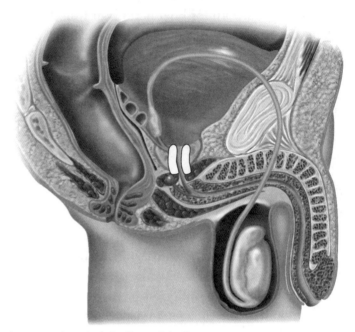

Figure 23 Location of collagen injection.
Data from American Medical Systems, Inc., Minnetonka, Minnesota (www.visitAMS.com).

each 4 weeks apart, are necessary. It is also possible that repeat collagen injections will be necessary over the long term. Collagen injections provide a continence rate of about 26% in postprostatectomy incontinence and a reduction in the number of pads used per day in an additional 37% of men.

The advantages of collagen injection are that it is minimally invasive, it is repeatable, it is associated with a short recovery period, and if it fails, it does not prevent you from pursuing other forms of therapy. Disadvantages of collagen therapy are that only a small percentage of men become totally dry, a small number of men develop a urinary tract infection, and 11% of men have transient urinary retention requiring clean intermittent catheterization. Permanent retention has not been reported.

Lastly, some individuals will experience transient dysuria (discomfort with voiding) and urgency after the procedure. The best candidates for collagen are men who have higher Valsalva leak point pressures (> 60 cm H_2O), who do not have overactive bladders, have not had prior radiation or cryotherapy, and who have not had a vigorous incision of a bladder neck contracture. With the advent of less invasive surgical options with better results, collagen is less frequently used.

Artificial urinary sphincter: The artificial sphincter is a mechanical device that is composed of a cuff that is placed around the urethra, a pump that is placed in the scrotum, and a reservoir that is positioned in the abdomen (**Figures 24** and **25**, page 202). All of these parts and the tubing that connects them are buried under the skin and are not visible. The cuff remains filled with sterile fluid and compresses the urethra. When you wish to urinate, the pump is pressed, and this transfers fluid out of the cuff, allowing you to urinate. The cuff automatically refills to compress the urethra. Placement of the artificial sphincter requires general or spinal anesthesia and an overnight hospital stay. Initially after the surgery, the sphincter is "deactivated" so that it doesn't work. It will be "activated" 4 to 6 weeks after surgery, when the tissues have healed and the swelling and sensitivity have subsided. The artificial sphincter achieves success rates of 80–85% regardless of the degree of incontinence. It is the most effective treatment for severe incontinence and for radiated patients. The sphincter can be used after collagen has failed. Disadvantages of the sphincter include mechanical malfunction rates of 10% to 15%, erosion rates of zero to 5%, and infection rates of 3%. Erosion is the migration of the device into another site. The cuff may erode into the urethra or through the skin,

Artificial urinary sphincter

A prosthesis designed to restore continence in an incontinent person by constricting the urethra.

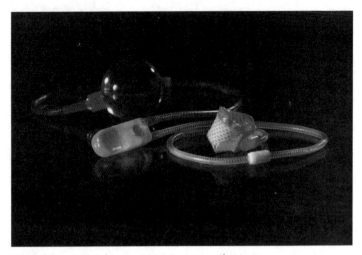

Figure 24 AMS Sphincter 800 urinary prosthesis.

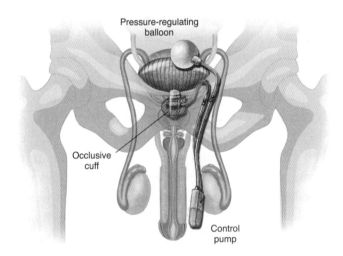

Figure 25 Location of artificial sphincter.

and other parts of the sphincter may erode into the skin or other areas. If there is an erosion, the device must be removed. Similarly, if the sphincter becomes infected, it must be removed. It is very important that a urodynamic study be performed before the sphincter is placed to make sure that the bladder holds an adequate amount of urine at low pressures and to identify an overactive bladder, which would require additional treatment.

Over time the pressure of the cuff on the urethra may cause the urethra to become thinner and the cuff to be less effective in compressing the urethra, requiring placement of another cuff in a separate area. Tandem cuff (2 separate cuff) models of artificial sphincters can be placed to minimize this from occurring.

Male slings: Slings have been used for some time in women with stress incontinence and have proven to be successful and durable procedures. Because of the success in women, they have been used more recently in men who are incontinent after radical prostatectomy. The sling may be derived from the patient's own tissues, from a synthetic (manmade) material, or from cadavers. The goal of the sling is to place tissue under the urethra to act as a buttress or a hammock. The tissue is anchored to either the abdominal wall or the pubic bone.

A variety of slings have been used to treat post-prostatectomy incontinence including a bone anchored sling, a **transobturator sling**, and a quadratically fixed sling. Slings that have been used for post prostatectomy incontinence in the United States include the Advance Male Sling System from AMS, which is a minimally invasive outpatient procedure. In other countries, the PROACT system (Uromedica, available in Europe), Remeex system sling (Neomedic, Barcelona), and Argus sling (Promedon, Argentina) are available.

Success rates in males with mild to moderate stress incontinence, post prostatectomy are comparable to the artificial urinary sphincter. With more severe incontinence, the sling is less efficacious. Complications

Male sling

A procedure to promote urinary continence in which a piece of tissue is placed under the urethra to act as a hammock or buttress.

Transobturator sling

A type of sling used to treat stress urinary incontinence in females and in men with post prostatectomy incontinence.

associated with the slings include acute urinary retention and perineal pain. Rare complications include urethral erosion and infection. Compared with the artificial urinary sphincter, slings have a lower risk of infection, erosion, and urethral atrophy.

PART SEVEN

Social Effects of Prostate Cancer

I don't have a job or insurance.
How can I get my prostate checked?

Are there support groups for men with prostate
cancer, and if so, how do I find out about these?

I've never thought of dying before, but now that
I have been diagnosed with prostate cancer, I think
about it and wonder if there are things that I should
be doing to prepare myself for the inevitable.

More . . .

93. I don't have a job or insurance. How can I get my prostate checked?

You should discuss prostate cancer screening with your primary care provider. Prostate cancer screening includes a PSA blood test and a DRE and a PSA level determination. If either of these are abnormal, your primary care provider will refer you to a urologist. If you do not have insurance you can check with your local hospital to see if there are any free prostate cancer screening services. The examining physician tells you whether he or she thinks your prostate feels suspicious and whether further evaluation by a urologist is recommended. You receive your PSA results by mail at a later time. If your PSA is elevated, you will be told that further evaluation is indicated, and you will be expected to make an appointment with a urologist for this. Often, this service is provided at your local hospital and may be advertised in the newspaper. If you have not seen advertisements in the past, you may want to call your local hospital to see if it is offered. If you are not able to obtain any information from your local hospital, you may want to try the offices of local urologists. If you plan to return to the free prostate cancer screening on a yearly basis, keep in mind that the same person may not examine your prostate each year and the PSA results from year to year may not be compared. For this reason, it is important that you keep track of the results and compare them yourself. Ideally, the PSA should not change by more than 0.7 to 0.75 ng/mL per year, even if each of the values is within the normal range. If the change is greater than 0.7 ng/mL per year, even if both numbers fall within the "normal range," then you should seek further evaluation. Transrectal ultrasound–guided prostate biopsies are not part of the free prostate cancer screening.

94. Are there support groups for men with prostate cancer, and if so, how do I find out about these?

Yes, there are prostate cancer support groups. These often can be found at your local hospital and meet on a regular basis. At our institution, they are held on a monthly basis. Often, there are guest speakers at the support groups to address key concerns of the group, such as nutrition, treatment of erectile dysfunction, treatment of urinary incontinence, and updates on newer forms of chemotherapy, in addition to group discussion time. Prostate cancer support groups provide an informal setting to express one's concerns, ask questions, and share information with others. Often, spouses and significant others attend and are invited to discuss their concerns. Discussing some of your concerns with others who are going or have gone through what you are experiencing may help alleviate some of your anxieties and help you focus on what questions you need to have answered by your doctor(s) as you make treatment decisions. To find out about your local prostate cancer support group, ask your urologist or your local hospital. The American Cancer Society (see **Appendix**) may also be able to help you identify a local prostate cancer support group.

95. I've never thought of dying before, but now that I have been diagnosed with prostate cancer, I think about it and wonder if there are things that I should be doing to prepare myself for the inevitable.

None of us like to think about our life ending, particularly if we feel healthy. Because we don't like to think about dying, we often do not prepare for it. All individuals, whether they are healthy or ill, need to think about death. End-of-life decisions, such as one's views on resuscitation measures and living wills, should be addressed long before one becomes ill. Financial issues and wills should be prepared and discussed with your family in advance. There is nothing more disheartening than for someone to become ill and not be able to make decisions, leaving the family at a loss as to what that individual would want. This is extremely important for measures like resuscitation, in the event that your heart stops, and other interventions to prolong life, such as nutritional support and ventilatory support (breathing machines). In addition, if you are in charge of the finances, it is important for you to identify one family member to discuss financial matters with early so that you may counsel that person as to how to manage the finances in your absence.

If you are unclear about what legal issues need to be addressed, it may be helpful to consult a lawyer. The American Cancer Society has a brochure that discusses more common things that need to be addressed, including questions regarding business, taxes, and loans. You will want to make sure that the following are in order and that you discuss them in advance with your family: life insurance, retirement plans, titles to assets, property, bank accounts, debts, safe deposit boxes, stock, car deeds, and will. It is important that beneficiaries are designated and that account numbers, addresses, telephone numbers, and contact people are recorded. All of this information should be in a location that is accessible to your family, and your family needs to know that you have taken care of these matters.

96. How will treatment of my prostate cancer affect my sexuality?

All forms of treatment of prostate cancer, with the exception of watchful waiting, have the risk of causing erectile dysfunction. Hormone therapy affects libido (desire for sex) in addition to erection function. But erectile function is only one part of your overall sexual function, and other phases of your sexual response can occur without a rigid penis. Sexual arousal can occur with other forms of stimulation and does not require penile rigidity. Orgasm also occurs in the absence of penile rigidity. After a radical prostatectomy, you have a dry ejaculate (no fluid will come out of the penis). The ejaculate volume may also be affected to varying degrees by interstitial seed therapy and EBRT.

It is very important to realize that your "sexuality" and your partner's sexual fulfillment are not lost because you can't achieve a rigid erection. Should you choose not to proceed with treatment for erectile dysfunction, you and your spouse or partner can still have a fulfilling sex life. It may require that you both re-address your own sensuality and what is stimulating for each of you and incorporate this into your sexual life. Thus, what is so often perceived as a "devastating" side effect of prostate cancer treatment can actually bring you and your spouse or partner closer together if both of you are willing to openly discuss sexual preferences, other forms of stimulation, and so on. Studies have demonstrated that many men are concerned that when they lose their erectile function, they are no longer a "man." On the contrary, women indicate that, in general, they do not think that this causes their spouse or husband to be any less of a man, and they indicate that other forms of intimacy, such as hugging, touching, and kissing, are just as important to them as sexual intercourse. Lastly, many women find that they are better able to achieve an orgasm with touching and finger stimulation than with vaginal intercourse.

Retreating and avoiding sex may only cause you more stress and anxiety. If you find it hard to discuss your sexuality and the changes that have occurred, then it may be helpful to seek out a specialist who can help you and your spouse adjust to the changes that have occurred in a more positive manner.

97. I've just found out that I have prostate cancer and I am depressed. Is this common?

Cliff's comment:

When you get the news, especially when there have been no warning signs and you are feeling great—to say that you may get depressed is an understatement. I had just recently retired, bought a beautiful home on a lake, and was looking forward to so many things; then I was told I have that horrible thing, CANCER. I became very anxious and depressed. My wife begged me to get some temporary medication while I was waiting to undergo the radical prostatectomy, but I refused. I was "too strong of a man" for that stuff—BIG MISTAKE! In the time it took for the results of my prostate biopsy to return and for me to undergo the radical prostatectomy, my blood pressure climbed significantly as a result of my anxieties. Instead of treating the underlying problem, I was given higher and higher doses of blood pressure medications. Well, that didn't help me and may have contributed to some of my problems in the postoperative period. Next time, I'll listen to my wife. An antidepressant to help me get through those few weeks before surgery would have been very helpful for me—I was a wreck, and it would have been nice to have had the help.

The diagnosis of prostate cancer comes as a shock to most men. Often, they are feeling fine and experience no signs or symptoms to make them suspicious. When they are faced with such a shock, common reactions are fear, anger, confusion, and depression. It is not unusual to initially "retreat" from life as you absorb the reality of the situation and begin to gather information and start the decision-making process. If you find that you have feelings of failure, are continuing to withdraw socially, feel that you are being punished, are thinking about committing suicide, feel helpless and can't make decisions, have lost interest in activities that brought you pleasure, or are crying a lot, then you may suffer from a more severe depression and you should discuss this with your doctor. Sometimes, when faced with such potentially overwhelming situations, you may need some assistance to help you gain control of your life again and make the decisions you will need to make regarding your treatment.

98. How will the diagnosis of prostate cancer affect me, my spouse/partner, and our relationship?

Cliff's comment:

I had just recently retired, bought a dream house on the water, and was thinking about the future. Finding out that I had prostate cancer and the acute realization that perhaps I did not have too long to live made me look critically at my future and my relationship with my family. Looking back, I realize how supportive my wife and family were throughout the whole ordeal. My wife helped me get over the initial shock, got me through the surgical recovery, and kept me thinking optimistically as I waited for my first PSA value after the surgery. My children also rallied on my behalf. My son stayed with me several nights in the hospital, which I realize must have been very difficult for him, as he is aware that he is at increased risk for prostate cancer.

I thank God each day for the blessing that he has bestowed on me. I live each day to the fullest. I am no longer putting things off to the future. I am very thankful that I will continue to be able to see my grandchildren grow up, and I take advantage of each opportunity that I have to be with my family. I feel that the stresses that I went through both before and after surgery and my family's support during this time have brought us all closer together.

Each individual is different, and each relationship is different, so it is hard to generalize about how each of you, and the two of you together, will react. In general, it appears that there are different aspects of prostate cancer and its treatment that are more stressful for you and your spouse or partner. Men generally appear to be most concerned with changes that are related to the treatment of prostate cancer, namely erectile dysfunction and urinary incontinence. Women, however, are more concerned about long-term survival. It appears that as couples face the challenge of dealing with prostate cancer, one of the critical steps is re-establishing their commitment to each other. This is achieved by open communication, which may be verbal or nonverbal, such as a hug. The absence of this sense of reconnection between partners, often as a result of failure of communication, can distance the relationship and make mutual support more difficult.

There is a delicate balance for couples between acknowledging fears that arise and keeping them private. Either extreme, being too vocal or too private, appears to create tension. Sometimes men do not express their worries and fears because they are concerned about the effect that this may have on their spouse. They often indicate that they have held things back because they didn't want to worry their spouses or felt that their spouses were not strong enough to deal with the issues. It is important that you communicate your concerns and fears with someone, whether it be your physician, close friend, relative, or men going through similar experiences, if you feel that you cannot discuss them with your spouse or significant other. Prostate cancer support groups, such as "Man to Man" or "Us Too," may be very helpful in this situation.

Confronting a life-threatening illness is difficult, but through open communication and mutual support, it can draw a family closer together, force a reordering of priorities, and influence a change toward a healthier lifestyle for all of those affected.

99. My husband/partner was just diagnosed with prostate cancer. What can I do to help him?

The diagnosis of prostate cancer can be devastating. Initially, shock and sadness are present, then once the shock has worn off, the decision-making process begins. Most men need to re-establish equilibrium, to get things back in order, as soon as possible. Taking an active role in the decision-making process tends to alleviate some of their anxieties. Men tend to be less vocal about their concerns and worries than women; whereas women tend to confide their concerns and worries to close friends and relatives, men often share this information only with their spouse or partner. You are indeed your husband's/partner's main, possibly only, support system, and this is very important to him. Your support, reassurance, and efforts in helping him acknowledge and cope with the diagnosis and treatment of prostate cancer will encourage him considerably. Studies have shown that married men with prostate cancer live longer than divorced, widowed, or single men with prostate cancer. It appears that this is related to the emotional support and possibly better health habits that married men have. Thus, helping your husband or partner maintain or optimize his health can be very important. Proper nutrition (see Question 17) and physical exercise will be of great benefit from both a physical and an emotional standpoint.

It is important to periodically reaffirm your commitment to the relationship and your partner/husband. Your awareness of your husband or partner's need to return to normal life as soon as possible and your willingness to facilitate this will help him greatly. Supporting your husband's efforts to seek help if he is feeling despondent and depressed is also important.

100. Will I be able to do the things I used to do now that I have prostate cancer? Can I travel? Can I golf?

Cliff's comment:

Since I had my radical prostatectomy, I can enjoy all of the things that I could before surgery. I am golfing and hiking and feel like my previous self. The only recognizable limitation was that I could not donate blood after treatment— one must be a cancer survivor for five years before they will accept my blood. As of January 2004, though, I can go to the local Red Cross facility and gladly donate a pint of blood to help someone else.

All forms of therapy may fatigue you for a few weeks after the procedure, but by one month after treatment, you should be back to full activity.

A lot of what you will be able to do will vary with the stage of your disease and the treatment that you are undergoing. With early-stage prostate cancer, there are usually few limitations; you can golf, travel, and so on. If you are planning to undergo surgical treatment, you will want to take good care of yourself before surgery. It is helpful to make sure that you are eating right, resting, and getting regular exercise.

There will be a recovery period after the surgery, and your doctor will indicate when he or she feels that you can resume full activity. The recovery period varies with the surgical procedure used. Recovery from the laparoscopic approach appears to be quicker than with the traditional open approach, and with interstitial seed therapy, the convalescence is much shorter than with surgery. If, however, you have trouble voiding after the procedure, you may require clean intermittent catheter-ization until the swelling in your prostate subsides. You can travel while performing clean intermittent catheter-ization; you just need to pack a catheter and the lubri-cating jelly. Radiation therapy takes several weeks to complete, and because it is performed 5 of the 7 days of the week, it requires that you "stay put" for a period of time. All forms of therapy may fatigue you for a few weeks after the procedure, but by one month after treatment, you should be back to full activity. If you are receiving the intramuscular form of hormone therapy and you wish to travel, you can make arrangements with urologists in the area to which you are traveling to get the shots. Often, your doctor can send a letter to the urologist in advance.

There are many organizations and publications that can provide you with more information. A list of many such resources is provided in the **Appendix**.

Appendix

Organizations

American Academy of Medical Acupuncture
www.medicalacupuncture.org
By Telephone: 323-937-5514
By Mail: AAMA, 4929 Wilshire Boulevard, Suite 428, Los Angeles,
California 90010

American Cancer Society
www.cancer.org
By Telephone: 1-800-ACS-2345
By Mail: American Cancer Society National Home Office, 1599 Clifton Road,
Atlanta, GA 30329
American Cancer Society Man to Man Support Groups
www.cancer.org/docroot/CRI/content/

American Foundation For Urologic Disease/Prostate Health Council
www.afud.org
By Telephone: 800-242-2383
By Mail: 300 West Pratt Street, Suite 401, Baltimore, MD 21201-2463

American Prostate Society
www.ameripros.org
By Telephone: 410-859-3735
By Fax: 410-850-0818
By Mail: 1340-F Charwood Rd, Hanover, MD 21076

American Society of Clinical Oncology
www.asco.org
By Telephone: 703-299-0150
By Mail: 1900 Duke Street, Suite 200, Alexandria, VA 22314

American Urological Association
www.AUAnet.org—clinical guidelines for the management of locally confined
prostate cancer 2007 guidelines

American Urological Association Foundation
By Mail: Patient Education 1000 Corporate Boulevard
Linthicum, MD 21090
By Telephone:
Toll Free (U.S. only): 1-866-RING AUA (1-866-746-4282)
Phone: 410-689-3700
Fax: 410-689-3800
www.auafoundation.org   www.urology health.org

Cancer Care, Inc.
www.cancercare.org
By Telephone: 212-712-8400 (admin); 212-712-8080 (services)
By Mail: 275 7th Avenue, New York, NY 10001

Cancer Research Institute
www.cancerresearch.org
By Telephone: 1-800-99-CANCER (800-992-26237)
By Mail: Cancer Research Institute, 681 Fifth Avenue,
New York, NY 10022

CaPcure (The Association for the Cure of Cancer of the Prostate)
www.capcure.org
By Telephone: 800-757-CURE or 310-458-2873
By Mail: 1250 4th Street, Santa Monica, CA 90401

Centers for Disease Control and Prevention (CDC)
www.cdc.gov
By Telephone: 404-639-3534
Toll Free Number: 800-311-3435
By Mail: Centers for Disease Control and Prevention, 1600
Clifton Rd., Atlanta, GA 30333

Department of Veterans Affairs
www.va.gov
By Telephone: 202-273-5400 (Washington, D.C. office)
Toll Free Number: 800-827-1000 (reaches local VA office)
By Mail: Veterans Health Association, 810 Vermont Ave., NW,
Washington, DC 20420

Health Insurance Association of America (HIAA)
www.hiaa.org
By Telephone: 202-824-1600
By Mail: 555 13th Street NW, Suite 600, East Washington, D.C. 20004-1109

Health Resources and Services Administration
Hill-Burton Program
www.hrsa.gov/osp/dfcr/about/aboutdiv.htm
By Telephone: 301-443-5656
Toll Free Number: 800-638-0742
800-492-0359 (if calling from the Maryland area)
By Mail: Health Resources and Services Administration,
U.S. Department of Health and Human Services,
Parklawn Building, 5600 Fishers Lane, Rockville, MD 20857

International Cancer Alliance (ICARE)
www.icare.org/icare
By Telephone: 800-ICARE-61 or 301-654-7933
By Mail: 4853 Cordell Avenue, Suite 11, Bethesda, MD 20814
By Fax: 201-654-8684

National Cancer Institute
www.nci.nih.gov
By Telephone: 301-435-3848 (Public Information Office line)
By Mail: National Cancer Institute Public Information Office,
Building 31, Room 10A31, 31 Center Drive, MSC 2580,
Bethesda, Maryland 20892-2580

National Center for Complementary and Alternative Medicine
nccam.nih.gov
By Telephone: 1-888-644-6226
By Mail: NCCAM Clearinghouse, P.O. Box 7923,
Gaithersburg, Maryland 20898

National Comprehensive Cancer Network
www.nccn.org
By Telephone: 888-909-NCCN (888-909-6226)
By Mail: National Comprehensive Cancer Network,
50 Huntingdon Pike, Suite 200, Rockledge, PA 19046

Prostate Cancer Organizations

Astra Zeneca Pharmaceuticals LP
www.prostateinfo.com

The Prostate Cancer Education Council
By Telephone: 800-813-HOPE, 212-302-2400
By Mail: 1180 Avenue of the Americas, New York, NY 10036

The Prostate Cancer Infolink
www.comed.com/prostate
By Mail: c/o CoMed Communications, Inc., 210 West
Washington Square, Philadelphia, PA 19106

**Prostate Cancer Research and Education Foundation
   (PC-REF)**
www.prostatecancer.com
By Telephone: 619-287-8860
By Fax: 619-287-8890
By Mail: 6699 Alvaro Rd, Suite 2301, San Diego, CA 92120

Prostate Cancer Resource Network
pcrn.org
By Telephone: 800-915-1001 or 813-848-2494
By Fax: 813-847-1619
By Mail: P.O. Box 966, Newport Richey, FL 34656

Social Security Administration
Office of Public Inquiries
www.ssa.gov
By Telephone: 800-772-1213
                800-325-0778 (TTY)
By Mail: Social Security Administration, Office of Public
Inquiries, 6401 Security Blvd., Room 4-C-5 Annex, Baltimore,
MD 21235-6401

United Seniors Health Cooperative (USHC)
www.unitedseniorshealth.org
By Telephone: 202-479-6973
Toll Free Number: 800-637-2604
By Mail: USHC, Suite 200, 409 Third St, SW,
Washington, DC 20024

US TOO International, Inc.
www.ustoo.com
By Telephone: 800-808-7866, 630-323-1002
By Fax: 630-323-1003
By Mail: 903 North York Rd, Suite 50, Hinsdale, IL
60521-2993

Web Sites with General Cancer Information

411Cancer.com
About.com (search on "cancer")
CancerLinks.org
CancerSource.com
CancerWiseTM/MD Anderson Cancer Center,
  www.cancerwise.org
National Cancer Institute's CancerNet Service,
  cancernet.nci.nih.gov/index.html.

Web Pages on Specific Topics

Alternative Therapy
Information on acupuncture: www.medicalacupuncture.org
(see American Academy for Medical Acupuncture).

Comprehensive web site about alternative therapies for cancer:
www.healthy.net/asp/templates/center.asp?centerid=23.

Chemotherapy
www.yana.org offers online and in-person support groups for
those going through high-dose chemotherapy.

Drug information for chemotherapy and hormonal therapy,
including information on financial assistance:
www.cancersupportivecare.com/pharmacy.html.

Clinical Trials
National Cancer Institute's CancerTrials site lists current clinical
trials that have been reviewed by NCI.

Coping

National Coalition for Cancer Survivorship (www.cansearch.org, 877-NCCS-YES) offers a free audio program, "Cancer Survivor Toolbox, including ways to cope with the illness. (Web site also has a newsletter, requiring yearly membership fee).

R. A. Bloch Cancer Foundation (www.blochcancer.org) offers an inspirational online book about cancer, relaxation techniques, and positive outlooks on fighting cancer, as well as trained one-onone support from fellow cancer patients.

Diet and Nutrition (Cancer Prevention)

USDA Dietary Guidelines: www.usda.gov/cnpp.

American Institute for Cancer Research provides tips on how to reduce cancer risk. www.aicr.org.

Cancer Research Foundation of America's Healthy Eating Suggestions: www.preventcancer.org/whdiet.cfm.

Family Resources

www.kidscope.org is a website designed to help children understand and deal with the effects of cancer on a parent.

Genetic Counseling

The National Society of Genetic Counselors web site (www.nsgc.org) lists society members, complete with specialty.

The National Cancer Institute has a searchable list of health care professionals who specialize in genetics and can provide information and counseling. http://cancernet.nci.nih.gov/genesrch.shtml.

Articles on genetics and cancer: http://cancer.med.upenn.edu/causeprevent/genetics.

Legal Protections, Financial Resources, and Insurance Coverage

The American Cancer Society offers a number of relevant documents to help understand your coverage, legal protections, and how to find financial assistance. Search http://www.cancer.org using keyword "insurance."

Medicaid Information: www.hcfa.gov/medical/medicaid.htm.

Family and Medical Leave Act:
www.dol.gov/dol/esa/public/regs/statutes/whd/fmla.htm.

Health Care Financing Administration's (HCFA) information
website about Breast Cancer and Medicaid programs:
www.hcfa.gov/medicaid/bccpt/default.htm.

www.needymeds.com offers information about programs
sponsored by pharmaceutical manufacturers to help people who
cannot afford to purchase necessary drugs.

www.cancercare.org/hhrd/hhrd_financial.htm offers listings of
where to look for financial assistance.

The National Financial Resource Book for Patients:
A State-by-State Directory: data.patientadvocate.org/.

Nausea/Vomiting
National Comprehensive Cancer Network:
www.nccn.org/patient_guidelines/nausea-and-vomiting/
    nausea-and-vomiting/1_introduction.htm.

Royal Marsden Hospital Patient Information On Line:
www.royalmarsden.org/patientinfo/booklets/coping/
    nausea7.asp#heading.

Treatment Locators: Physicians and Hospitals
AIM DocFinder (*State Medical Board Executive Directors*):
www.docboard.org/.

Nonprofit organization providing a health professional licensing
database.

AMA Physician Select (*American Medical Association*):
www.amaassn.org/aps/amahg.htm.

AMA database of demographic and professional information on
individual physicians in the United States.

American Board of Medical Specialties: provides verification of
physician qualifications and has lists of specialists.
www.abms.org/, 1-866-ASK-ABMS or American Board of
Medical Specialties, 1007 Church Street, Suite 404,
Evanston, IL 60201-5913

Approved Hospital Cancer Program (*Commission on Cancer of the American College of Surgeons*):
www.facs.org/public_info/yourhealth/aahcp.html

The Approvals Program of the Commission on Cancer surveys hospitals, treatment centers, and other facilities according to standards set by the Committee on Approvals, which recommends approval awards in specific categories based on these surveys. A hospital that has received approval has voluntarily committed itself to providing the best in diagnosis and treatment of cancer. Approved hospitals can be searched by city, state, and category.

Association of Community Cancer Centers: Cancer Centers and Member Profiles:
www.accc-cancer.org/members/map.html

Geographic listing of ACCC members with contact information, and description of cancer program and services *as provided by the member institutions.*

Best Hospitals Finder (*U.S. News & World Report*):
www.usnews.com/usnews/nycu/health/hosptl/tophosp.htm.

The *U.S. News* hospital rankings are designed to assist patients in their search for the highest level of medical care. Database is searchable by specialty, including the top cancer hospitals (www.usnews.com/usnews/nycu/health/hosptl/speccanc.htm) or by geographic region.

Best HMOs Finder (*U.S. News & World Report*):
www.usnews.com/usnews/nycu/health/hetophmo.htm
U.S. News guide to choosing a managed-care option.

HMOs and Other Managed Care Plans (Cancer Care):
www.cancercare.org/patients/hmos.htm
Discusses the advantages and disadvantages of HMO care.

Hospital Select (*American Medical Association & Medical-Net, Inc.*):
www.hospitalselect.com/curb_db/owa/sp_hospselect.main

Hospital locator database searchable by hospital name, city, state, or zip code. Hospital Select data include basic information (name, address, telephone number); beds and utilization; service lines; and accreditation.

National Cancer Institute Designated Cancer Centers: cancertrials.nci.nih.gov/finding/centers/html/map.html

Directory of NCI-designated Cancer Centers, 58 research-oriented U.S. institutions recognized for scientific excellence and extensive cancer resources. Listings feature phone contact numbers, website links and a brief summary of website resources.

National Comprehensive Cancer Network (NCCN): www.nccn.org

The NCCN is an alliance of leading cancer centers. NCCN members (www.nccn.org/profiles.htm) provide the highest quality in cancer care and cancer research. NCCN offers a patient information and referral service (www.nccn.org/newsletters/1999_may/page_5.htm) that responds to cancer-related inquiries and provides referrals to member institutions' programs and services (1-888-909-6226).

Physician Qualifications

The American Board of Medical Specialities www.abms.org; click on "who's certified" button (search by physician name or by specialty).

Radiation Therapy

National Cancer Institute/CancerNet: Radiation Therapy and You: A Guide to Self-Help During Cancer Treatment cancernet.nci.nih.gov/peb/radiation/. By phone, free of charge: 1-800-4-CANCER (in English and Spanish).

Books and Pamphlets

The following pamphlets are available from the National Cancer Institute by calling 1-800-4-CANCER:
- "Chemotherapy and You: A Guide to Self-Help During Treatment"
- "Eating Hints for Cancer Patients Before, During, and After Treatment"
- "Get Relief From Cancer Pain"
- "Helping Yourself During Chemotherapy"
- "Questions and Answers About Pain Control: A Guide for People with Cancer and Their Families"

- "Taking Time: Support for People With Cancer and the People Who Care About Them"
- "Taking Part in Clinical Trials: What Cancer Patients Need to Know"

Available in Spanish:
- "Datos sobre el tratamiento de quimioterapia contra el cancer"
- "El tratamiento de radioterapia; guia para el paciente durante el tratamiento"
- "En que consisten los estudios clinicos? Un folleto para los pacientes de cancer"

The following pamphlets are available from the National Comprehensive Cancer Network:
- "Prostate Cancer Treatment Guidelines for Patients"
- "Cancer Pain Treatment Guidelines for Patients"
- "Nausea and Vomiting Treatment Guidelines for Patient with Cancer"

Available in Spanish:
- "Cáncer de la próstata"
- "El dolor asociado con el cáncer"

Carney KL, 1998. *What is Cancer Anyway? Explaining Cancer to Children of All Ages.*

Hapham WH, 1997. *When a Parent Has Cancer: A Guide to Caring for Your Children.*

Landay, D, 1998. *Be Prepared: The Complete Financial, Legal, and Practical Guide for Living with a Life-challenging Condition.*

Glossary

#

4K score: Determined by levels of total PSA, free PSA, intact PSA, and human kallikrein 2 — helps improve diagnostic accuracy for clinically significant prostate cancer.

A

Active surveillance: A form of prostate cancer therapy whereby no definitive treatment is instituted initially, but definitive therapy is instituted when predefined changes are noted.

Acupuncture: A Chinese therapy involving the use of thin needles inserted into specific locations in the skin.

Adrenal glands: Glands located above each kidney. These glands produce several different hormones, including sex hormones.

Agent Orange: A herbicide containing trace amounts of a toxic chemical dioxin that was used during the Vietnam war to defoliate areas of the forest.

Alopecia: Partial or complete loss of hair from parts of the body where it normally grows (baldness).

Alpha blocker: An alpha adrenergic receptor blocker used to treat benign prostatic enlargement.

Alternative medicine: The treatment is used instead of accepted treatments.

Androgen deprivation therapy (ADT):
A treatment based on the reduction of androgen hormones, which stimulate prostate cancer cells to grow.

Androgen receptor blocker: A chemical that binds to the androgen receptor preventing the binding of androgens (testosterone and dihydrotestosterone).

Androgens: Hormones that are necessary for the development and function of the male sexual organs and male sexual characteristics (i.e., hair, voice change).

Antiandrogen: A medication that eliminates or reduces the presence or activity of androgens.

Artificial urinary sphincter: A prosthesis designed to restore continence in an incontinent person by constricting the urethra.

Asthenia: Abnormal physical weakness or lack of energy.

Avanafil (Stendra): A phosphodiesterase type V inhibitor used to treat erectile dysfunction.

B

Benign: A growth that is not cancerous.

Benign prostatic hyperplasia (BPH): Noncancerous enlargement of the prostate.

Biomarker: A characteristic that is objectively measured and evaluated as an indicator of normal biological processes, pathologic processes or pharmacological responses to a therapeutic intervention.

Biphosphonate: A type of medication that is used to treat osteoporosis and the bone pain caused by some types of cancer.

Bladder neck contracture: Scar tissue at the bladder neck that causes narrowing.

Bladder outlet: The first part of the natural channel through which urine passes when it leaves the bladder.

Bone scan: A specialized nuclear medicine study that allows one to detect changes in the bone that may be related to metastatic prostate cancer.

Bound PSA: PSA attached to the proteins in the bloodstream.

Bowel preparation: Cleansing (and sterilization) of the intestines before abdominal surgery.

Brachytherapy: A form of radiation therapy whereby radioactive pellets are placed into the prostate.

BRCA1: Gene which may increase the risk of prostate cancer.

C

Cancer: Abnormal and uncontrolled growth of cells in the body that may spread, injure areas of the body, and lead to death.

Castrate-resistant prostate cancer (CRPC): Prostate cancer that is resistant to hormone therapy and resultant low (< 20 ng/dL) testosterone level.

Castration: The removal of both testicles.

Catheter: A hollow tube that allows for fluid drainage from or injection into an area.

Catheterization: The insertion of a hollow tube that allows for fluid drainage from or injection into an area.

Cell: The smallest unit of the body. Tissues in the body are made up of cells.

Chemotherapy: A treatment for cancer that uses powerful medications to weaken and destroy the cancer cells.

Clean intermittent catheterization: The placement of a catheter into the bladder to drain urine and the removal after the urine is drained at defined intervals throughout the day to allow for bladder emptying. It may also be performed to maintain patency after treatment of a bladder neck contracture or urethral stricture.

Clinical trial: A carefully planned experiment to evaluate a treatment or medication (often a new drug) for an unproven use.

Coapt: To close or fasten together.

Collagen injection: Injection of a chemical around the urethra that compresses the urethra and bladder neck to help treat stress urinary incontinence.

Colostomy: A surgical opening between the colon (large intestine) and the skin that allows stool to drain into a collecting bag.

Complication: An undesirable result of a treatment, surgery, or medication.

Confirm MDx: Special gene test that uses DNA methylation to detect likelihood of prostate cancer on a repeat biopsy.

Conformal EBRT: EBRT that uses CT scan images to better visualize radiation targets and normal tissues.

Cryotherapy, cryosurgery: A prostate cancer therapy in which the prostate is frozen to destroy the cancer cells.

CYP17: An enzyme in the adrenal gland and testes that is needed for testosterone production and other chemicals.

CYP17 inhibitor: An inhibitor of the CYP17 enzyme in the testes and adrenal glands, which is needed for testosterone production.

Cystoscope: A telescope-like instrument that allows one to examine the urethra and inside of the bladder.

D

Decipher: 22 gene based test that predicts the likelihood of high-grade prostate cancer and metastatic disease after radical prostatectomy.

Deep venous thrombosis (DVT): The formation of a blood clot in the large deep veins, usually of the legs or in the pelvis.

Diethylstilbestrol (DES): A form of the female hormone estrogen.

Doubling time: The amount of time that it takes for the PSA level to double.

Dysuria: Painful urination.

E

Ejaculation: The release of semen through the penis during orgasm. After radical prostatectomy and often after a TURP, no fluid is released during orgasm.

ELAVL1: RNA binding protein that may have a role in prostate cancer progression.

Epidural anesthesia: A special type of anesthesia whereby pain medications are placed through a catheter in the back, into the fluid that surrounds the spinal cord.

Erectile dysfunction: The inability to achieve and/or maintain an erection satisfactory for the completion of sexual performance.

ExoDx prostate intelliscore urine exosome assay: Score based on 3 genes (ERG, PCA 3, SPDEF)—helps determine risk of Gleason 6, 7, and benign disease on initial prostate biopsy.

F

Fistula: An abnormal passage or communication, usually between two internal organs, or leading from an internal organ to the surface of the body.

Flare reaction: A temporary increase in tumor growth and symptoms that is caused by the initial use of GnRH agonists. It is prevented by the use of an antiandrogen 1 week before GnRH agonist therapy begins.

Fluoroscopy: Use of a fluoroscope, a radiologic device that is used for examining deep structures by means of X-rays.

Foley catheter: A latex or silicone catheter that drains urine from the bladder.

Food and Drug Administration (FDA): Agency responsible for the approval of prescription medications in the United States.

Free PSA: The PSA present that is not bound to proteins. It is often expressed as a ratio of free PSA to total PSA in terms of percent, which is the free PSA divided by the total PSA × 100.

Frequency: A term used to describe the need to urinate often.

G

Gastrointestinal: Related to the digestive system and/or the intestines.

General anesthesia: Anesthesia which involves total loss of consciousness.

Gland: A structure or organ that produces substances that affect other areas of the body.

Gleason grade/score: A newer technique to stratify prostate cancer risk, 5 categories.

Gleason scale: A commonly used method to classify how cells appear in cancerous tissues; the less the cancerous cells look like normal cells, the more malignant the cancer; two numbers, each from 1 to 5, are assigned to the two most predominant types of cells present. These two numbers are added together to produce the Gleason score. Higher numbers indicate more aggressive cancers.

GnRH antagonist: A form of hormone therapy that works at the level of the brain to directly suppress the production of testosterone without initially raising the testosterone level.

Gonadotropin-releasing hormone (GnRH) agonists: A class of drugs that prevent testosterone production by the testes.

Granulocyte macrophage colony-stimulating factor (GMCSF): A protein secreted by several cells that stimulates the growth and development of various cells.

H

Hemibody: Half of the body.

Hernia: A weakening in the muscle that leads to a bulge, often in the groin.

Hesitancy: A delay in the start of the urine stream during voiding.

Hormones: Substances (estrogens and androgens) responsible for secondary sex characteristics (hair growth and voice change in men).

Hormone therapy: The manipulation of the disease's natural history and symptoms through the use of hormones.

Hot flushes: The sudden feeling of being warm, may be associated with sweating and flushing of the skin, which occurs with hormone therapy.

Hypocalcemia: Low calcium level in the bloodstream.

Hypoechoic: In ultrasonography, giving off few echoes; said of tissues or structures that reflect relatively few ultrasound waves directed at them.

Hypogonadism: In males, a condition in which the testes do not produce enough testosterone.

Hypokalemia: Low potassium level in the bloodstream.

I

Immune response: The response of organs, tissues, blood cells, and substances that fight off infections, cancers, or foreign substances.

Immunotherapy: The treatment of disease by inducing, enhancing, or suppressing an immune response.

Incision: Cutting of the skin at the beginning of surgery.

Infarct: An area of dead tissue resulting from a sudden loss of its blood supply.

Intensity modulated therapy (IMRT): An advanced form of 3D conformal radiation.

Intermittency: An inability to complete voiding and empty the bladder with one single contraction of the bladder. A stopping and starting of the urine stream during urination.

Interstitial: Within an organ, such as interstitial brachytherapy, whereby radioactive seeds are placed into the prostate.

IsoPSA: A new test that is based on the fact that molecules (proteins) produced by cancer cells have different 3D structures than the same proteins produced by normal cells. Still under investigation.

L

Laparoscopic radical prostatectomy: Removal of the entire prostate, seminal vesicles, and part of the vas deferens via the laparoscope.

Laparoscopy: A surgical procedure in which a fiber-optic instrument is inserted through the abdominal wall to view the organs in the abdomen or to permit a surgical procedure.

Lymph: A clear fluid that is found throughout the body. Lymph fluid helps fight infections.

Lymph node(s): Small, bean-shaped glands that are found throughout the body. Lymph fluid passes through the lymph nodes, which filter out bacteria, cancer cells, and toxic chemicals.

Lymphocele: A collection of lymph fluid in an area of the body.

M

Male sling: A procedure to promote urinary continence in which a piece of tissue is placed under the urethra to act as a hammock or buttress.

Malignancy: Uncontrolled growth of cells that can spread to other areas of the body and cause death.

Medical oncologist: See **oncologist**.

Metastases: Deposits of prostate cancer outside of the prostate and lymph nodes.

Metastatic castrate-resistant prostate cancer (mCRPC): Prostate cancer that continues to progress despite ADT and castrate levels of testosterone and has spread to sites outside of the prostate, commonly the lymph nodes and bones.

Morbidity: Unhealthy results and complications resulting from treatment.

Mortality: Death related to disease or treatment.

Multifocal: Found in more than one area.

N

Neoadjuvant therapy: The use of a treatment, such as chemotherapy, hormone therapy, and radiation therapy, before surgery.

Nerve-sparing: With regard to prostate cancer, it is the attempt to avoid damaging or removing the nerves that lie on either side of the prostate gland that are in part responsible for normal erections. Injury to the nerves can cause erectile dysfunction.

Nocturia: Awakening at night with the desire to void.

Noninvasive: Not requiring any incision or the insertion of an instrument or substance into the body.

Nucleotide: Any of various compounds consisting of a nucleoside combined with a phosphate group and forming the basic constituents of DNA and RNA.

O

Occult cancer: Cancer that is not detectable through standard physical exams; symptom-free disease.

Oncogene: A gene that in certain situations can turn a cell into a cancer cell.

Oncologist: A medical specialist who is trained to evaluate and treat cancer.

Orchiectomy: Removal of the testicle(s).

Osteoblastic lesion: Pertaining to plain X-ray of a bone, increased density of bone seen on X-ray when there is extensive new bone formation due to cancerous destruction of the bone.

Osteoclast: A specialized cell that breaks down bone.

Osteolytic lesion: Pertaining to a plain X-ray of a bone, refers to decreased density of bone seen on X-ray when there is destruction and loss of bone by cancer.

Osteonecrosis of the jaw (ONJ): A severe bone disease that affects the bones of the jaw, maxilla, and mandible. It may occur in association with bisphosphonate and RANK-ligand inhibitor use.

Osteoporosis: The reduction in the amount of bone mass, leading to fractures after minimal trauma.

Overflow incontinence: The involuntary loss of urine related to incomplete emptying of the bladder.

P

Palliative: Treatment designed to relieve a particular problem without necessarily solving it; e.g., palliative therapy is given in order to relieve symptoms and improve quality of life, but it does not cure the patient.

Palpable: Capable of being felt during a physical examination by an experienced doctor. In the case of prostate cancer, this refers to an abnormality of the prostate that can be felt during a rectal examination.

Paresthesia: Abnormal sensation, typically tingling or prickling, that could be due to nerve damage.

Pathologist: A doctor trained in the evaluation of tissues under the microscope to determine the presence/absence of disease.

Pelvic floor muscle exercises: Exercises that help one strengthen muscles that aid in the control of urinary incontinence.

Penile clamp: A device placed around the penis to prevent urine leakage.

Penile prosthesis: A device that is surgically placed into the penis which allows an impotent individual to have an erection.

Percutaneous: Through the skin.

Performance status: An attempt to quantify cancer patients' general well-being and activities of daily life.

Perineal prostatectomy: Removal of the entire prostate, seminal vesicles, and part of the vas deferens through an incision made in the perineum.

Perineum: The area of the body that is behind the scrotum and in front of the anus.

PHI: See **Prostate health index**.

Prostatic intraepithelial neoplasia (PIN): An abnormal area in a prostate biopsy specimen that is not cancerous, but may become cancerous or be associated with cancer elsewhere in the prostate.

Placebo: A fake medication ("candy pill") or treatment that has no effect on the body that is often used in experimental studies to determine if the experimental medication/treatment has an effect.

Positive margin: The presence of cancer cells at the cut edge of tissue removed during surgery. A positive margin indicates that there may be cancer cells remaining in the body.

Posterior: The rear or back side.

Prednisone: A synthetic (manmade) drug that is similar to corticosterone.

Priapism: An erection that lasts longer than 4 to 6 hours.

Prognosis: The long-term outlook or prospect for survival and recovery from a disease.

Prolaris: Uses a score based on level of expression of mRNA of 31 cell cycle progression genes and 15 housekeeping genes. Associated with risk of death and metastatic disease.

Prostate-specific antigen (PSA): A chemical produced by benign and cancerous prostate tissue. The level tends to be higher with prostate cancer.

Prostatic acid phosphatase (PAP): An antigen produced by prostate cancer cells.

Progression-free survival: The length of time during and after treatment during which the disease being treated (cancer) doesn't progress (get worse).

Prostate health index (PHI): A mathematical formula that relies on differing proportions of specific biomarkers—can be helpful in distinguishing between benign prostatic hypertrophy (BPH) and prostate cancer.

PSA nadir: The lowest value that the PSA reaches during a particular treatment.

PSA velocity: The rate of change in PSA over time.

R

Radiation oncologist: A physician who treats cancer through the use of radiation therapy.

Radiation therapy: Use of radioactive beams or implants to kill cancer cells.

Radium 223: A radioisotope administered intravenously for the treatment of bone metastases.

RANK-ligand inhibitor: A chemical that binds that prevents RANK-ligand from functioning.

Retention: Difficulty in emptying the bladder of urine; may be complete, in which one is unable to void, or partial, in which urine is left in the bladder after voiding.

Robot-assisted radical prostatectomy: A radical prostatectomy performed with the assistance of a robot.

S

Salvage: A procedure intended to "rescue" a patient after a failed prior therapy, e.g., a salvage radical prostatectomy after failed external-beam therapy.

SCHLAP1: Potential biomarker for the determination of risk of prostate cancer metastatic progression.

Select MDx: Urinary 2 gene assay (HOX 6 and DLK1) used to identify high grade prostate cancer.

Semen: The whitish fluid that is released during ejaculation.

Seminal vesicles: Glandular structures that are located above and behind the prostate. They produce fluid that is part of the ejaculate.

Sensitivity: The probability that a diagnostic test can correctly identify the presence of a particular disease.

Sensory neuropathy: Damage to the nerves of the peripheral nervous system that can cause abnormal sensations, like tingling or a prickling feeling.

Stendra: See **Avanafil**.

Stomatitis: Inflammation of the lining of the mouth.

Stress incontinence: The involuntary loss of urine during sudden rises in intra-abdominal pressure, e.g., with coughing, laughing, sneezing, or picking up heavy objects.

T

Taxane(s): A chemotherapy drug derived from the yew tree that prevents cell growth by inhibiting special cell structures, called microtubules, which are involved in cell division.

Testis: One of two male reproductive organs that are located within the scrotum and produce testosterone and sperm.

Testosterone: The male hormone or androgen that is produced primarily by the testes and is needed for sexual function and fertility.

Testosterone replacement therapy (TRT): The practice of giving testosterone to treat conditions in which the testes do not produce enough testosterone.

Thrombocytopenia: A decrease in the platelet count of the blood.

TMPRSS2-ERG: A prostate specific gene which is an oncogene for prostate cancer. In combination with PSA and PCA3 it provides improved accuracy in diagnosing prostate cancer.

TNM System: The most common staging system for prostate cancer. It reflects the size of the tumor, nodal disease, and metastatic disease.

Total (maximal) androgen blockade: The total blockage of all male hormones (those produced by the testicles and the adrenal glands) using surgery and/or medications.

Transobturator sling: A type of sling used to treat stress urinary incontinence in females and in men with post prostatectomy incontinence.

Transperineal: Through the perineum.

Transurethral prostatectomy (TURP): A surgical technique performed under anesthesia using a specialized instrument similar to the cystoscope that allows the surgeon to remove the prostatic tissue that is bulging into the urethra and blocking the flow of urine through the urethra. After a TURP, the outer rim of the prostate remains.

Tumor: Abnormal tissue growth that may be cancerous or noncancerous (benign).

U

Unit: Term referring to a pint of blood.

Upper respiratory tract infection: An acute infection involving nose, sinuses, and throat.

Ureters: Tubes that connect the kidneys to the bladder, through which urine passes into the bladder.

Urethra: The tube that runs from the bladder neck to the tip of the penis through which urine passes.

Urge incontinence: The involuntary loss of urine associated with the urge to urinate and is related to an overactive bladder.

Urinary incontinence: The unintentional loss of urine.

Urologist: A doctor that specializes in the evaluation and treatment of diseases of the genitourinary tract in men and women.

V

Vaccine therapy: A type of immune therapy which involved the injection of a chemical into an individual.

Vas deferens: A tiny tube that connects the testicles to the urethra through which sperm passes.

Vasectomy: A procedure in which the vas deferens are cut and tied off, clipped, or cauterized to prevent the exit of sperm from the testicles. It makes a man sterile.

W

Watchful waiting: Active observation and regular monitoring of a patient without actual treatment.

Z

Zones: An area of the prostate distinguished from adjacent areas.

Index